Beth Am...
Enjoy
in time
Michael Myers
7-3-20

The Ancestor

The Ancestor

Michael Meyer

XULON **PRESS**

Xulon Press
2301 Lucien Way #415
Maitland, FL 32751
407.339.4217
www.xulonpress.com

Author's Coach: Jacqueline Arnold, www.sweetlifeusa.com

Printed in the United States of America.

ISBN-13: 978-1-54562-814-0

Dedication

Dedicated to my mother Bette Meyer, and her
parents Mr. and Mrs. John Miller, and to her
sisters Patricia, Janis, and Gwynna for preserving
my heritage with memorable stories.

Table of Contents

Dedication v
Introduction ix

The Ancestor 1
Far From My Home 3
Something's Missing 11
Are You Happy? 17
Losing Control 21
Find Him 25
A Soldier's Grave 31
The Letter 37
Somewhere In Time 43
A Rebel Soldier's Dying Wish 49
A Question Of Sanity 55
The Quantum Equation 59
Andersonville 65
Looking For Answers 75
Tick Tock 83
Finding Sarah 89

I Own A Plantation 95

Mourning Sonata. 109

A Slave's Bounty. 117

General Sherman and The Letter 133

Sarah's Nightmare. 137

Brunch With Sherman. 143

The Hunting 159

Sarah's Dilemma. 169

Thanksgiving, God and Country 179

Alter The Past 187

Dancing Miss Sarah 193

Covered In Blood 199

Daniel Surrenders 203

The Map 207

A Child Is Coming. 213

We're Going In! 219

Last Stop Andersonville 225

The Sting. 237

Bring Out Your Dead 261

Daniel Summary 267

Diary Of An Ancestor 273

Glory Hallelujah! 281

Providence Spring. 287

References and Influences 289

Michael Meyer, Author, Family Historian 293

Introduction

With death comes new life - that's called ancestry. It is the origin or descent of someone or something. An accurate knowledge of one's ancestry can enhance the significance of your past and give purpose to your present and future. Millions of Americans would love to know their heritage, but, unfortunately few can trace their past more than one or two generations to discover its richness.

I've been fortunate to have been handed down not only the knowledge of my family's lineage, but also what I consider a treasure trove of letters, documents, diaries, photographs and relics – tangible evidence of my family's ancestry which has enabled my imagination to weave a fictional story, based on historical fact.

My mother, Bette Meyer, and her parents, Mr. and Mrs. John Miller, were the keepers of my family's history, and preserved our ancestry, and the relics belonging to my great-great-grandfather, a soldier in the bloodiest clash on U.S. soil – America's Civil War (1861-1865).

My great-great-grandfather, James H. Miller, a Sergeant in the Union Army, died a horrible slow death in Andersonville Prison - the worst prison in American history, which became infamous for the horrific, gruesome deaths of more than 13,000 Union Civil War soldiers.

He was young, handsome, wholesome, and hopeful that the war would soon be over so he could be with his "Dear affectionate wife," Rachel Emma Miller, who was with child during their separation. According to letters written to his wife, and eventually handed down to my mother, he had been camped with the 31st Regiment Illinois Volunteer Infantry along the "Big Black"- part of a campaign in Mississippi that lay idle during winter months.

In his letter dated February 2, 1864, he indicated to his wife that he felt "movement astir." Unfortunately, it was his last letter home, for according to another letter from the Regiment's Captain to his wife, he went missing on February 29th, 1864, had not been seen, and was presumed captured by the "Rebs."

February; coincidentally, the exact same month of the opening of the gates of hell, known as Andersonville Prison. Surviving just four months in the prison's squalor, it was recorded that he died June 21, 1864 – sadly, just three weeks after the birth of his child he never saw, my ancestor and great-grandfather, James. A. Miller. Their names separated by only a middle initial, their lives forever entwined in my family tree. Yes, the cycle of life is the law of nature – and with death comes new life.

To add to this sorrow, which was prevalent during that period, Rachel died a little more than three-and-a-half years later, in January 1868, leaving her child, James A. Miller, to be raised by her brother, Charles Orr, or "Uncle Charlie Orr," as my family affectionately called him.

Uncle Charlie also served in the Civil War as a Union soldier. As good fate would have it, he wrote a journal and memoir chronicling his own exploits during the Civil War with the 52nd Illinois Infantry Regiment, from the Battle of Shilo to Sherman's March to the Sea.

"Mud, mud, mud," he would write of that rainy winter and Georgia's swampy, red earth terrain, which he and 60,000 other troops had to endure.

Today the South is better appreciated because of its beautiful layers of carved-out rural countryside and some preserved buildings, towns, and cities, to be enjoyed only because of the modern conveniences of transportation, air conditioning and heating. Back then, the harsh elements and red Georgia clay and mud seemed so foreign to a Northern soldier. One was to have said in his diary "this is the stupidest country God ever made."

I have delved deep in to these family records with great interest. All of Charlie Orr's recollection and journal entries match the historical records I have researched. Many a soldier after the war died from chronic wounds, disease, hardship, or poverty, with some just plain giving up to the brokenness of spirit. I believe that child who was left to his care – James A. Miller, gave my great-great uncle Charlie the determination to do whatever it took to carry on in life to a ripe old age, and as a result, perpetuate the family line. Through Rachel's death, he received the gift of new life, which yielded for him both significance and purpose.

My mother, the granddaughter of that child, was born Bette L. Miller in 1925, in Stillwater, Oklahoma. Her parents, Mr. and Mrs. John Miller, would settle in rural Kansas, where I would later spend some of my summers and my high school years, transplanted from the contrasting big city life in which I was being raised, in southern California.

Those visits created fond memories for me, and afforded me the small-town, 'Norman Rockwell America' experience in Garden City, Kansas, before the franchise modernization came. The changing seasons, cruising main street, wheat fields in the breeze, a distant train whistle late at night, meeting friends at the local soda fountain shop, stealing a kiss on that first warm summer night, I was living the life of the Saturday Evening Post magazine, which was actually delivered to my grandfather's porch like clockwork every weekend morning. To add to this simple life, were the unforgettable family reunions, where many family members gathered every year, featuring tables laden with homemade cooking, the heavy scent of elderly perfumes, and colored with afternoon stories of relatives come and gone. Reunions were for meeting friendly and sometimes cute cousins, culminating with evenings at the piano and fiddle medleys, singing church hymns and prairie tunes. This was my heritage; warm feelings from times spent together with family were etched in my heart and mind, and planted in my DNA.

It was also here at my grandparents' house that I discovered, tucked away in the basement, a "secret" closet every boy dreams of – that hidden treasure and mystery of days gone by. Relics from the 1800's - a weight scale for gold, a photograph campaign pin of Abraham Lincoln, a tintype leather photo album, and among all the items, what really stood out was a Civil War sword and leather sheath. My eyes grew like saucers when I stumbled upon this treasure. I could only imagine the stories it could tell. This well-preserved family heirloom would later become the fulcrum of my passion and purpose to sit and write today.

My grandfather died in 1988, leaving my mother to care for his home and wife until she died in 1998. My mother made sure I ended up with the sword, as she was the oldest daughter, and I the oldest of cousins. It was my grandfather's request to pass them on and to leave the trail of history for others in the family.

My mother's sister and many cousins had made their homes in Georgia. My mother ended up choosing a retirement community in the South to be near her family so she could enjoy regular visits from them. When I would come visit my mother from California, I would pester her about 'that storage unit piled with junk' and chastise her about wasting her money. She insisted on keeping it.

In 2003, my wife Barbara and I bought a second home in Fayetteville, Georgia, in order to be near my mom and also, my wife's family in nearby Tennessee. It was Barbara who turned me on to her Southern ways, traveling in the South and soaking up her many stories of growing up in the hills of Tennessee. Memories of papa's moonshine still, momma's make-do cooking, the unbelievable poverty, hunting for 'bar' meat (bear), teaching me what a 'toe sack' is and how it's used in so many ways, and getting lost on a pig trail.

Soon after moving here, mother died in 2004 after several months of complications following surgery. During that period of her convalescence, mom shared with me a vivid dream she recalled about a boy, the identity of the child was unknown to her. At her funeral, I was told by my son that I was going to be a grandfather. And, to our surprise, the baby was a boy. Perhaps, my mother's vivid dream was a glance of future life. So, with death, comes new life.

After her funeral, I would soon sort through that storage unit of hers that I had long complained about – and, to my great discovery, buried beneath all the junk, was an old metal box. Initially, I simply shelved it for a rainy day. Then, one fall day, three years after her death, I opened it, and found a treasure trove of letters, diaries, and photographs that no one in our family had known about. I can't imagine my life without having discovered these cherished memories – for me, it was like finding a Monet! Thank you, mom.

These family treasures were a deep connection to my family heritage and also bridged the gap and ignited my interest in the history of our country, the Civil War, and the role my family members played in it. The cost of death and sacrifice our ancestors paid to give each new generation a better quality of life, promised to us in our founding documents of life, liberty, and the pursuit of happiness, was only made richer by the family relics and treasures now in my possession.

During the Civil War, the high casualty rate in one battle alone, a Union victory of sorts - at Antietam, (Sharpsburg, MD), gave birth to the Emancipation Proclamation. The horrific blood-soaked fields and hills of Gettysburg, (PA), which became a turning point in the war, resulted in what is considered to be the finest speech given by an American President, The Gettysburg Address. Then the South succumbed to the death nail at the Fall of Atlanta (GA), and yet, delivered new life and assurance to the re-election of Abraham Lincoln, which yielded the 13th Amendment and the preservation of the United States of America. All told, the deaths of over 750,000 soldiers, with millions of wounded men, including their broken wives and families, gave new life and freedom, and not only preserved our union, but added hope to every black American to this day. The cost of battle is high, but the family roots run deep, and the horrific deaths give way to new life.

Every family relic, every letter and photo tells a story that unravels the mysteries of the past. Searching for clues to the answers of the 'Who, What, Where, When, How and Why, is in our DNA. Everyone loves a good mystery and searching out the truth and the answers that unlock the mysteries of our existence.

Our DNA has a lot of those answers. It gives us a glimpse of our story, our family tree, our roots, and is one way to piece together the puzzle, scientifically. If you add history, soft science and theory to the mix, along with some fictional and non-fictional characters, a dash of romance, a pinch of plot twists, and a big surprise or two, then hopefully it's enough to serve up an adventurous recipe that keeps you wanting another taste. In other words, you'll want to turn the page to find out what happens next - a journey in time that reveals a family mystery.

And this is the plot of the story I am about to share. Based on the truths I discovered from my family tree, incorporated into fictional characters to develop an interesting story; I will take you on an adventure of war and romance, poverty and prosperity, death and life, the wonders of time and portals of time, and the mystery of The Ancestor.

First, I pose a few appetizer questions to intrigue you, dear reader.

Does God really intervene in the affairs of mankind? How is this relevant to today? What if you could go back in time, would you? Would you try and alter history? What time period would you chose? Would you explore your family roots or the history of our nation? Is today's civil unrest simply repeating history?

Why did the Civil War last years instead of months? Were pride and ego factors in an extended war? Why did 13,000 men die a horrible death in Andersonville prison in less than a year? Was there purpose for this and did it serve the war effort? What was the reason they stopped exchanging prisoners? How could this happen in America? Who is the real Ancestor?

Have you ever considered your family story? If you don't know, then imagine one; ask questions of your family, dig for buried treasures and search for answers in your basements and your attics, around your family table, and through family heirlooms from days gone by.

In the meantime, enjoy mine - they've finally been given a voice.

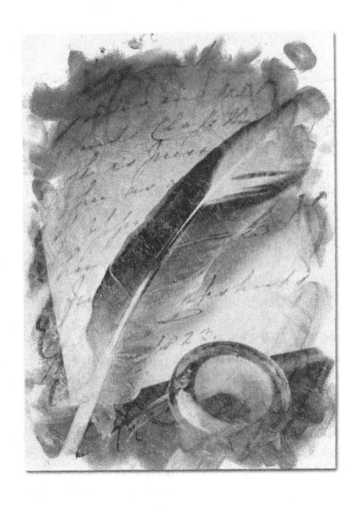

The Ancestor

F all crisp leaves blow across a long-retired graveyard –
moving slowly toward a particular granite stone.
    Imagine the soft voice of a young female with a unique
English accent in poetic cadence.

"Sometimes when the wind blows the autumn leaves
across the graves,
I can hear the calling of our fore bearers
Their journeys and longings, the pains of war,
Along with the fallen brave
Such Days of glory and nights pass with vintage wine
The seed of children planted, grown, blossom in time
Their lanterns gone out now just granite stones waiting
for the name
Is life only for hollow ground to be forgotten?
Left meaningless, such a shame
Oh, dreaded fear of death without purpose
An end to a life so full the sky so clear
The faceless trees are bending now
Their voices are drawing me near
To hear the stories the graves ignore
My only prayer they hear my verse
And that I be remembered as The Ancestor."

The name inscribed on the old gravestone reveals:

Rachel Emma Montgomery
March 7, 1832 - January 12, 1868

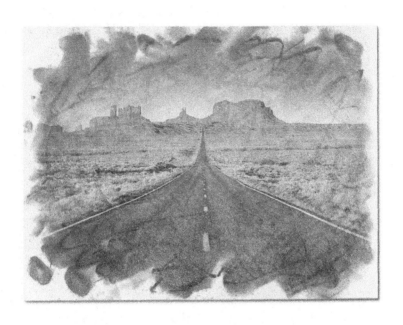

Far From My Home

From a bird's-eye view, a black Lexus SUV is driving a straight, long highway toward a sloping hill through New Mexico under a crisp sun. Absorbed somewhere else, Daniel is talking to his excitable publishing agent in California, while he continues driving uphill in the middle of nowhere.

Daniel has just turned 50, slightly silvered and dark haired, somewhat tall with attractive features. He blends his humor with most experiences, yet he's sensitive when called upon.

"Daniel, what do you mean you're driving to Georgia? You had plane tickets. You're kidding, right?"

Daniel looks at his odometer and then takes a quick glance at his fuel gauge. The sign ahead warns: <u>Next Gas, 90 Miles</u>.

"I'm just outside Gallup," he notes his position to the demanding voice on the other end of the phone, "I need this time to myself. You'll get that story Jason."

Jason, on the other end of the phone connection, is standing by a large office window in a Los Angeles high-rise overlooking the hustle and bustle of a never-ending city, with a piping hot Starbuck's in hand.

"Let me guess," Daniel says dryly, "Peruvian Dark Roast with two shots of espresso."

"The deadline Daniel. Don't leave me hanging. Please. And, it's three shots," Jason retorts.

"Have I ever?" Daniel disconnects the call and continues down the long highway, drifting in thought. Time passes without any boredom.

Just before dark, Daniel starts looking for a prairie motel on the outskirts of Amarillo. He's not the marathon driver like his father, as he recalls from his childhood. Memories flood his mind of a time when he traveled this familiar Route 66 as a boy passenger, watching every iconic scene flash by as he was looking out his window. He floats in between reality and memories.

Even then, his imagination was creating life-like stories. He was always intrigued by the remoteness of an endless desert yet colored with those lone diners, retro motels, and village towns he'd pass in the blink of an eye, wondering who could possibly live such an isolated life. Those giant billboards every few miles were like watching a preview to a strange upcoming freak show of giant rabbits, towering Dinosaurs, rattlesnake catchers, and Ol' Chief Yellow Horse who could sell just about anything to anyone.

That had all changed now; I-40 had become a major highway with little trace of that bygone era. He pulls in to the only motel he has seen for miles. It's nothing like the big city he has come from, but it's got a vacancy blinking on the neon road sign. It will do for one night of accommodations and it looks clean enough.

Daniel is up early the next morning, leaving the outskirts of Amarillo while listening intently on his cell phone to his wife, "I understand Daniel, but the way you left, and so distant. I was hoping we'd sleep together before you left. My time is right *now*," A petulant female voice demands from the other end of the call.

"Michelle, I left early to drive and think. You know my feelings about children. We've discussed this," Daniel was irritated and reluctant to address this subject yet again.

Back in Los Angeles her silhouette appears near a window. She flops on her back on the yielding bed, sighing, "But a child, it's what I have long dreamed of. I'm willing to forgo my career. We need a change Daniel." She was not relenting, and yet, there was no meeting of the minds.

"I know," is all he can muster. The road ahead yields a panoramic view to a wide-open space. Daniel seems so remote from his surroundings, and from the Michele he married seven years ago.

Just before crossing Arkansas into Tennessee, Daniel gets out and stares at the bright sun through his shades. He aches and stretches, then enters a quaint motel lobby and notices the TV on the wall blaring. It's a news report with a brilliant shot of the sun. A national reporter covering a story somewhere in middle America flashes across the screen.

"These unusually high solar flares are said to be the cause disrupting weather and power grids, not only locally, but around the globe. Reports are coming in of strange phenomena. Our science advisor..." the reporter's voice trails off as Daniel turns to the clerk who fades the television sound into the background with a hand-held remote.

"You pulled in just in time," the well-tanned clerk assured Daniel. "Bad storms in the direction your headed." He gives a nod to the television and the recent report.

Daniel was glad to be off the road again, having driven many more miles than anticipated today and glad to be away from the leash of the cell phone. It was now recharging in his new motel room for the night.

Daniel sits on the bed and stares, not opening his bags. He hears the voice of his mother's doctor in his head and his last words. "*Your mother will be fine Daniel. We perform this operation routinely, anymore. It's just an extra precaution that we asked you to be here."*

They were starting to haunt him as he replayed the doctor's words over and over again trying to make sense of it all.

After a bagel breakfast at the motel and some inadequate coffee, Daniel crosses the bridge over the Mississippi into Memphis while conversing with his mother.

"Yeah mom, I drove," he says, shrugging it off, "I should be there soon. How are you feeling?"

"Tired," she says in a very sluggish way, "Wishing I could do more."

"I do too, mom," Daniel empathizes. "Mom...I'm staying...I mean, for a while. I'll be looking at houses."

Those words just came out of his mouth, even surprising himself. The idea had been developing along the way but just finalized after hearing her voice. He can afford to be impulsive, which he's managed to keep under control, a lifestyle he's prided himself in maintaining. He wraps up his call feeling good about his decision, then continues through the transitioning, tree covered south, with its the starkly covered landscape of kudzu vines growing everywhere for miles upon miles of driving.

Alas, Georgia! Daniel arrives midday, cruising through the heart of Dixie, viewing old barns and abandoned farms, with no lack of churches, some new, but mostly aged with nearby cemeteries, weathered and fading into the overgrowth of nature. To Daniel, Georgia seems an endless sea of Pine and Magnolia trees, with no visible horizon in any direction. There's an occasional plantation-style home aside still lakes, both large and small, with horses grazing in open fields divided by rivers with bridges needing repair. He slows down to caution signs observing both black and white workers laboring side-by-side along the road. Daniel passes a sign indicating Dayton County. He drives up a winding road through a rural subdivision with two large houses seemingly out of place. It appears like the development just came to a halt. He then turns into the driveway of a property with a distinguished frontage and lush foliage, completely standing out from the rest.

The Greek revival, antebellum-style home, has obviously been remodeled to fit a modern, more contemporary estate. A middle-aged appealing female, dressed professionally and exuding Southern hospitality, greets Daniel as he approaches the porch.

Welcoming him is Miss Fitzgerald, whom he met and spoke with during his last motel stay near Memphis, where she vividly described which area she just so happened to originate from and could not stop talking about during their conversation. Her voice and Southern accent reminded him of some character from a Tennessee Williams play – a part she played quite well.

"Welcome to Georgia, Mr. Coffee."

"Daniel is fine," appreciating the cordialness.

"Mr. Daniel. You've had quite a lengthy drive. Would you care to relax a moment? I've set out a pitcher of tea and some lemon in the sun room." He doesn't have a chance to answer. "Of course, unless you're anxious to survey the property. You've arrived on a perfect day to get a feel for this lovely manor." The words roll off her tongue so smoothly as if she were born to sell property.

Daniel, in his normal nonchalant manner, is keenly observant of his surrounding, but especially of her charm. If authentic, which he had no reason to doubt, she was a pleasant change compared to the metropolitan personality of get in, get it done and get on to the next big thing. Yet, he was anxious, eager to simmer down and meld into the gentile landscape. He was seeking a change, for what, he didn't quite know. Something he'd hoped to accomplish without the usual conflicts, twists and turns the characters in his books had to go through in their quest for a happy ending.

Daniel looks about the manor grounds after her suggestion and then into her eyes, "I appreciate the offer. Perhaps after you show me around."

"Well then, let's start with the Great Room."

After surveying the inside, they walk out on the deck and view the overlook, with a sloping view down to a well-defined creek, where you can see the sun sparkling off the water. A forest of Evergreen, Pine, and Poplar trees stretched above the manor, but standing higher were a pair of giant twin Oaks, placed just right at either end of the structure. Their stature, age, and strength seem to keep guard of the house with pride.

"This is much better than I imagined," Daniel observes.

Miss Fitzgerald smiles, and slightly begins a closing performance with her Southern accent, "It deserves the care and attention that I see in your eye, Mr. Daniel. I know you will be a good caretaker. Why, I vision you writing a novel back here."

"Oh, I assure you Miss Fitzgerald, I am here strictly on sabbatical and to get my mother through recovery. Buying a house is, well, a second thought, a temporary accommodation and an investment, rather than impose on family during my extended stay. I'm not unpacking my laptop, and I'm even considering tossing this phone. I just want to get away from that L.A. pace to unwind and get centered - at any cost. This place seems ideal for that."

"Then you're in the right place Mr. Daniel. Why, time here just stands still when the wind blows just right."

Suddenly the breeze picks up and the trees gently voice their response by shimmering in the sun and slightly swaying. It's almost fall. Daniel looks out to the tree line, then back at her.

"I'll take it."

Something's Missing

Daniel's mother is slowly folding her clothing and putting items in a single overnight bag. She takes a picture of Daniel and Michelle from a dresser, pauses to look at it, then wraps it carefully in a small cloth and places it in the bag. The doorbell rings at her quaint, but stylish apartment.

"Mom?" she hears, knowing before announced who it is at her door ringing the bell.

Daniel doesn't need her to open the door, he has his own key and uses it to enter - he was just giving her ample warning, so as not to catch her off guard.

"In here Daniel," she calls in a slightly raspy voice.

He appears in her bedroom doorway; a look of such fondness quickly crosses his face as his eyes light on his beloved mother. He walks toward her ready for her welcome arms, "Mom."

They hug. Their mutual joy is evident. She's elegantly dressed, as usual, even when she is casually attired. If there's any gray in her auburn hair, it's unnoticeable. Her slender boned hands are now the most notable. In her younger days, her attractive features were such deep brown eyes, glamour looking hair, and her uncommonly shaped lips. He never thought of his mother as being petite but inside the embrace, he felt a small, fragile frame. He inherited his humor from her which was liable to pop up and surprise one at any moment, but now was not the time. There was something deeper inside of this embrace, as they slowly unwrap from one another.

"You look well. You're not tired of driving?" she asked as any mother would.

He looks at her packing items on the bed when he notices a book by a competing author and picks it up. "Just hungry, but please don't fix anything." He picks up other books and frowns, adding, "I'll eat out. What's this?" half kidding, he rather scolds her. "You're not taking one of my books?"

"Oh, I always loan yours out and they never seem to bring them back," she dismisses him.

"Where's Michelle?"

He looks at her with surprise then replies, deflecting her intent for honesty "You know how her work goes. She sends her wishes."

"She's a busy lawyer, I know. I was so hoping to see her walk in holding a baby. She'd be such a good mother - she'd slow down her career then."

He changes his demeanor slightly. "Mom, you know it's me. I told you both going in that wasn't in my future. My DNA isn't wired for fatherhood... caring, the time it takes... I'm driven by other things."

She stands up straight. "Daniel, she would've come if you'd asked her. Now she's confused. What's really wrong?"

He's now highly annoyed. "She called you?" He hesitates, then surrenders to his mother's familiar intuition.

"I'm in a strange place. I feel like I'm living in two worlds. When you make plans for the future and they all happen, well now what? More plans? More goals? Then watching it all go by. Success was great for a while but now, it all feels rather empty, like overnight, I woke up and something was missing."

She walks away into the living room listening as he follows. "Some wine?" she offers.

He pauses, with some relief, having expressed this unfamiliar feeling. "Yes, Please. That hasn't changed has it mom?"

She pulls out two wine glasses and hands him a bottle from her rack and a cork screw.

"It's not Michelle. I love her, but, it's like I can't see her. That life, the spark, it's not there. She's connecting, but I'm not. So, I decided to take some time, get some space between me and the L.A. madness."

"You mean run." She turned and looked at him wryly.

Plunk. The cork makes a thud as it pops out of the bottle and changes the atmosphere of silence.

He pulls out the cork screw then pours for both. She sips. He acknowledges her point with a gesture, toasting to her and then he takes a drink. Then another quick one to finish it. They sit readying for a conversation as she lights a cigarette.

"You keep making plans for the future, perhaps, what you're missing is in your past?"

He pours another drink for himself, listening.

She begins to wisely reflect, "You know, your father - those brave men, came home after the war and had it so good. The life of the future was theirs for the taking. It was all in those wonderful magazine ads and TV commercials. The suburban homes, the fancy two cars in every driveway, the promise of wonderful career opportunities, family, and of course, we housewives had all the luxurious modern inventions for the home that left us so much free time." She looks down as her fingers rub her wedding ring. "Precious time."

Daniel smiles a bit. "And you gave so much of it to me."

She takes a drag and exhales. "But your father wasn't happy. The war kept haunting him. Of course, he would never talk about it, so one day I asked him. He teared up and said, "Why me?" "Excuse me?" I said. "Why was he alive and all his buddies left scattered in the graves across Europe?"

She has Daniel's full attention, her body language shifting as if her husband were present, and continued reflecting with her vivid recollection. "Well, I was a bit taken by surprise, but it made sense. Here he was alive and living the American dream, but his soul was back there with his comrades in arms. An indescribable bond. So, it struck me. Did the others, his army friends, have those same thoughts? Of course, being men," she chuckles half-heartedly, "in that era, they didn't mention it to one another."

She stands and walks over to the mantle and takes a picture of a group of men with her husband pictured in it, front and center. She hands it to Daniel.

"I always wondered who these guys were with dad."

She smiles looking with fond memory. "They took my suggestion and all went back to Europe. As it turns out, they did have those same feelings, so off they went like a band of brothers and came home with the answer."

He looks up with expectation "Which was?"

"I can't tell you what's deep in the soul of a man, but he was changed. They all were."

Daniel hands back the picture "So, you're saying what I'm missing is…"

"He lived the rest of his life with a great sense of purpose. He died with no regrets."

Daniel looks away "I couldn't begin to give a child what you and dad have given me."

She breaks the poignant moment and jokes, "Well for heaven's sake, give the child to me then. I'll raise 'em."

Daniel stands and hugs her then he looks behind her and notices her cigarette has fallen from the ash tray to the floor. He swiftly reaches down to put it out, then looks at her.

"Mom," he says with serious concern, "I want you to come live with me. I bought a beautiful home, you can recover while I take care of you. That would give me purpose."

The phone rings. She reaches for it.

"You are out of your head. Hello?" she turns to grimace at the thought of losing her independence, "Doctor, oh yes," She smiles at Daniel. "He's here now. He and my sister will be bringing me."

Daniel casually wanders around. He sees a photograph of his mom and her sisters as little girls with her parents. There's a very old man with white hair and white beard sitting beside all of them. She hangs up.

"Doctor just wants a quick conference with you at the hospital before I go under."

"Why have I never seen this?" Daniel inquires, nodding in agreement.

She looks at it. "I've been going through storage and framing one at a time. There's a treasure of artifacts and letters I want to show you."

"Who's the much older man in the photograph, Mom?"

"That's your great grandfather. He was born during the Civil War. His father died at Andersonville Prison. That's what I was going to ask you. If you'd go through all those letters in my storage and find his story. I even think there's a diary somewhere."

He sets the picture down then ponders it a moment as she walks into the bedroom.

In time, mom, in time. Right now, I just need you to get through this.

Are You Happy?

At a nearby Waffle House Daniel is greeted by a choir of voices behind the counter and cook's station as he walks in.

"Welcome to Waffle House."

"Two up, no onion, medium," calls out the one waitress.

Daniel sits at the counter. An attractive black waitress in her late 30's – early 40's, approaches with a pot of coffee.

"Can I get you some coffee?"

His eyes roam around the Waffle House and his keen sense of observation begins to kick in. He thought he'd lost that sense, or was becoming numb to it in the bustling metropolis of unconscious movement, which he left behind. A fear of becoming 'just like them' was slowly being jarred free. *Maybe I am alive,* he thought.

The waitress asks again, "Some coffee for you?"

He takes off his sunglasses and sets them on counter then notices her name tag. The activity and chatter subside as he eyes her perfect, dark ebony skin.

"Sure, Donna," he smiles warmly, "Smells great. We don't have Waffle Houses in California."

She pours hot steaming coffee and smiles, "What brings you here?"

Daniel no longer can think or speak casual conversation, so he just puts it out there. "Are you happy?"

She hesitates then goes along with it, scoping out this obvious newcomer. "I try to stay busy and not think about it."

"Me, too," he agreed, glad to have a comrade in his numbness of life. "You said it exactly. Now I know why I'm here. I was looking for time to think about it. Thank you, now I can eat."

She smiles and makes light of the moment as he glances at the menu.

"Can I get you a happy meal, then?" They both laugh.

"All right, so, I'm too serious. I'll take a patty melt with hash brown and a sweet tea."

"That's all we have is sweet tea."

He grabs a paper left at the counter as she calls out his order.

The front-page headline reads: SUN FLARES DISRUPT POWER AND COMMUNICATION

He is intently reading the article, when what seems moments later, she brings his order. "Can I get you anything else?"

"This is fine, thank you."

He scarfs it down. After reading a bit more he leaves money at the counter and heads outside.

Donna steps outside from behind the counter calling, "Sir."

Just as he is about to open his car door, Daniel turns back noticing she's holding his sunglasses.

"You left your glasses." She gives a warm smile as she hands them over.

"Daniel. I'm Daniel. I'll probably be coming here a lot."

She pauses. "Please do, Mr. Daniel."

He drives off to continue his important errands of the day, watching her go back inside to his new favorite breakfast spot.

A short time later, inside a large, elegantly decorated furniture showroom, Daniel signs a check with a salesman who's just hung up the phone. Daniel's obviously tired from making several selections of furnishings for his new residence.

"We've scheduled delivery first thing in the morning," the salesman proudly declares.

Daniel disrupts emphatically "No, no! Afternoon. I have to take my mother for surgery in the morning."

"No problem. I'll let them know."

Later that evening, the sun sets beautifully behind the tall trees and outside Daniel's bedroom window as he's on his phone. "Are you sure you want this operation mom? Your age... there are other treatments for this type of cancer." He sighs, "I understand. See you in the morning." The power line noise is humming outside his open window. He shuts off his phone then settles into his makeshift bed on the floor.

The lights flicker, then stay off. Now it's quiet. Behind the house under the balcony deck area, strange noises begin moving across the fallen leaves.

Losing Control

The movers arrive at first light and are actively unloading furniture into the house. Daniel is pacing in the yard on his cell, a bit frantic.

"Look, Aunt Margret..."

His mother is standing at the door of her apartment about to leave. Her sister, Aunt Margret, is on his mother's phone. "Oh, Daniel, hello."

"I'm so upset right now. The movers are here at the wrong time. I can't leave right now..."

"Oh, don't worry, we were just on our way out the door."

"I'll be right there as soon as..."

She glances at his mother, "We'll just see you at the hospital. We'll be fine."

"Aunt Margret..." Daniel realizes she's hung up. Then he sees the phone installer pull up to connect the land lines.

"Why not everybody show up?" he verbalizes with exasperation. "It's only my mother!"

The installer steps out of his van wearing a fully equipped belt "Hey, looks like I'm just in time. Busy as hell, but I've got you covered. You lost cell service too?"

Daniel shakes his head 'no' like, what's he talking about?

"Solar activity. Cell towers are freaking out. Where do you want the land line?"

"Bedroom, kitchen, and living room," Daniel waves him inside.

The installer walks into the house so Daniel decides to try and relax, hoping he will be quick. He walks to his back acreage looking over the natural beauty. His eyes stop at the creek and he notices something on the ground. Leaning closer, he starts brushing away a layer of caked dirt and twigs. Closer examination reveals an antique pocket watch with a cracked crystal. The hands have stopped. He reaches carefully to scoop it up and holds it closer.

CRACK! The sound of a breaking branch startles him. Looking up, he sees a deer staring at him from across the creek. The animal, blending in the natural background, moves slowly, crunching the leaves and brush. Just then, Daniel's cell phone rings.

The phone display indicates it's his agent. Irritated that this moment of peace is invaded by outside forces determined to defeat his escape, he reluctantly takes the call, feigning as a matter- of- fact tone.

"Jason. I was just thinking about you. What timing," Daniel says flatly while he stares at the watch, then carefully places it in his pocket.

"I get it - you need time, so I got you an extension. What are agents for?"

"Oh, I don't know, lunch at Spago's?"

"Funny. Here's the deal, I just need the story...ahh synopsis. Gimme a couple of those great plots you weave and I'll stop bothering you."

"You're such a con, Jason," Daniel says wryly. "Okay, so you stop calling...it's about..."

Immediately, the phone starts emitting a loud, screeching static sound. He pulls the phone away from his ear, grimacing, and then holds it back to his ear.

"What's that strange noise? Can't hear you... hello?" quizzes Jason.

Daniel looks at the screen and sees the phone's clock is spinning wildly in time. Daniel yells into the phone at Jason through the confusion, "It's a story about a man who loses all contact with the outside world and is paranoid his agent is stalking him."

He then turns and throws the phone into the creek a few yards away. He quickly turns around and runs into the mailman standing right in front of him.

"Welcome to Summerville, Mr. Coffee. Sheila told me you bought this place. Just wrote a check and moved in. That's some way to live. You L.A. folks crack me up."

Daniel still a bit startled, looks back at the creek area where he threw the phone, then back at the mailman. "Yeah, we can be a bit impulsive. Who's Sheila?"

"The realtor."

"Oh yes. Fitzgerald, Ms. Fitzgerald."

With admiration, the post man admits, "I read a lot, especially fiction. I find your books most absorbing, especially the crime mystery. Your detective fella, attentive to detail yet somewhat aloof, goes by intuition more than fact."

"Ames. Inspector Ames."

"I must have missed your last book or two."

"Probably not, it's been a couple of years. Is that mail for me?"

The mailman holds out a book with a pen "Not really, I was hoping for an autograph Mr., Coffee."

"Daniel."

While Daniel signs the book thrust before him, he's wondering if he's in Mayberry and this is Barney Fife. Not in a condescending way, but, things are beginning to feel surreal.

"I'll be sure and make certain your mail arrives promptly, I know about deadlines," the mailman chuckles, but looks as if he is taking this job very seriously.

"I appreciate that..."

"Henry."

"Henry."

"So, Sheila gave you the history about this place? Wonderful lore...my favorite legend is the..."

"I'm sorry Henry, right now I have to attend to other matters and get to the hospital. My mother's going in for surgery."

"Oh, by all means. I hope it's not serious." Daniel walks with him around to the front. "Well, hope your power stays on. Most of the area is experiencing black outs right now."

A husky mover approaches Daniel as Henry returns to his mail vehicle.

"If you'll just sign here, then let us know where to place your furniture, we can finish up in a jiffy," he said in his good 'ol boy manner and accent. Daniel signs the delivery receipt.

"Yes sir, we moved your neighbor across the way, JJ Bynum. Boy, does he have some fancy bar and entertainment theater."

"He from around here?" responds Daniel trying to blend in.

Mover looks at him strange. "JJ? He's huge, a big-time basketball star. Always havin' parties and women hangin' all over 'em. He's got over 40 cars somewhere."

Daniel looks up the slight hill and skims the driveway of his neighbor's house and notices a Rolls and an exotic convertible. A flag pole with some type of iconic flag is waving in the breeze. Daniel feels a stir of panic; he is used to being the one in control. His heart starts fluttering. Confusion sets in. *What am I doing here?*

Find Him

It's now late afternoon at the Atlanta hospital and the doctor is talking with Aunt Margret outside a room. "We're concerned about her breathing. She seems to be struggling, so we may have to put her on a ventilator."

"She seems so weak. When can she talk?" Her sister Margret asks looking tired but concerned.

Daniel hurries in and finds her with the doctor. "Aunt Margret!"

They hug. Margret is slightly younger than her sister Gloria, and seemingly much livelier for her years. Widowed herself, but with a larger family that keeps her occupied. Her son, who is seated, talking on the phone, gives a slight wave to Daniel.

"This is Dr. Haggard," Aunt Margret makes the introduction. "She's having breathing problems."

Daniel holds out his hands and they shake.

"Not to worry, now. This happens sometimes with patients her age," the Dr. says calmly.

"The operation?"

The doctor looks at his chart. "So far it seems to have been the correct diagnosis. Give me a moment to confer with the other surgeons."

"Can I see her?" Daniel is getting anxious.

The doctor gestures to her room. Daniel and Aunt Margret enter and find she's being tended to by a nurse while sleeping and on tubes. Monitoring machines are consistently beeping.

"Poor thing," consoles Margret. "Bless her heart."

Daniel is not comfortable. "I should've been here. It's why I came all this way!"

Margret takes her hand and rubs it affectionately. Daniel stands near her bed while Margret straightens a vase of flowers, and then looks at her watch. "It's good that you're here now. Daniel, could you stay with her? It's been a long day and..."

"No, no. You go ahead. I can't thank you enough."

Aunt Margret smiles, then lovingly replies, "Don't forget, she's my darling sister too."

Daniel takes a seat and watches her lay there. Time passes. He falls asleep in the chair.

"Daniel," a weak voice calls.

He opens his eyes. "Mom?"

"You remember when you were a little boy and you played soldiers?"

Daniel's wondering if she's coherent, but agrees to soothe her.

"Yes mom, you let me hold a real old sword."

"I want you to have it. It was your great, great grandfather's in the Civil War."

He's teary-eyed. Choking up, he softly says, "Mom, don't talk that way."

She tries to reach for her water on her bedside but he grabs it for her and helps her sip through a straw.

"He's maybe the reason you're a writer. He wrote such beautiful letters to his wife."

Daniel watches her start to close her eyes then sits down and lays his head on her bed and starts back to sleep. More time passes. It's 3 AM.

"Daniel," she says, "Find him."

The clock on the wall stops. Aunt Margret enters the room somewhat later and relieves Daniel.

"Go home. Get some sleep." Daniel agrees, reluctantly, and leaves his mom's care to her sister.

It's barely past sunrise as Daniel lies sound asleep on the lounge chair on his deck. There's someone yelling from below who disturbs him, causing him to rise abruptly. Daniel pops up and sees it's Margret's son.

"It's cousin, Rick. Mom's been trying to call you," he shouts out with urgency. "Better get to the hospital right away. It's not good!"

Daniel arrives at the hospital and sees his aunt with family members. She's sobbing.

"Oh Daniel, I'm so sorry." She grabs him tight as Daniel turns white. "She passed holding my hand. Her soul is with God."

His world starts spinning as he almost falls. A nurse calls for assistance. Daniel is grabbing his chest around his heart when he suddenly shuts down and falls to the floor in a blackout.

When Daniel becomes conscious he is lying in a sterile room, staring up at the ceiling. The nurse is removing him from a heart monitoring machine. He has no sense of awareness of any time lapse.

The attending physician speaks to his situation with concern, "You're having strange, erratic signals from your heart."

"Arrhythmia," Daniel replies with a blank stare.

The physician looks surprised at Daniel's medical terminology. "Yes, arrhythmia, you've heard that before from your physician or…"

"I'm a writer. I research. It's a malfunction of the heart's electrical system," he recites, still with a glazed look.

"That's an excellent way of putting it. Your ECG can tell us a lot but not everything. "However," he glances at the printout in his hands, "you're either superhuman or an alien species. These readings…" the Dr. hesitates.

Daniel looks a bit more attentive. "These readings… what?" Daniel then looks around and asks, "Where am I anyway?"

Now the nurse and physician look at each other. She is careful with her wording, "We found you passed out on the floor…after you were informed…" she hesitates. "How much do you recall about your mother?"

"That's the last I do recall. I'm sorry, I barely know my name. I'm seeing things in strange color. What were you saying about my heart?" Daniel strains to be present.

"Are you on any medication? Had any issues before with your heart?"

"No, I'm very healthy. Why do I feel so… disoriented?" he struggles to find how he feels.

"My poor dear man, that's a tremendous loss you just suffered," the nurse interjects.

The Dr. tries to clarify, yet he himself seems baffled. "You're in some sort of shock yet, in a limbo state…"

"Limbo, that's it. That's how I feel. In limbo." Daniel sits up and buttons his shirt.

"We'll need to run some more tests and I need to get clarification on these arrhythmia readings," urges the Dr.

Daniel then stands up. "No. I need to go," he mumbles in a haze then looks at the monitor's last reading on the screen. "Could I get a copy of those?"

"We have grief counseling..." the nurse starts writing down some numbers.

Daniel's not listening as the Dr. hands him the chart pages and she hands him the numbers.

"I must go. Make arrangements and... just disappear. You know, arrhythmia limbo," Daniel concludes in his own way of making light of a serious but confusing situation when not in control, especially of his mental faculties, which he's never experienced in his life.

A Soldier's Grave

A lone cemetery that barely caught Daniel's eye when he first arrived just a few days earlier, becomes the setting of a chapter in his life he didn't see coming. Now it's the final home of his mother; as he's attending an unexpected funeral, and experiencing a shift in reality. Daniel and Michelle are thanking family and friends after the burial ceremony at her grave. Daniel slips away and walks slowly about 100 feet away to a group of much older grave sites.

Aunt Margret takes this moment to point out her observation to Michelle. "He has always been such a sensitive boy. His mother mentioned he seemed so distant…so numb. This was before she passed, on the way to the hospital."

A noticeably troubled Michelle agrees, "I just want my husband back. That sensitive boy I married. Aunt Margret, have you noticed? He hasn't even cried yet."

"Now that you mention, no, I haven't. Michelle, be patient. He'll return."

"And I'll be waiting with open arms. There will be no surrender here. Tell me, how are you holding up?"

In the distance, Daniel stoops down to one grave in particular. A dead confederate soldier's stone. The marker reads:

BELOW LIES A CONFEDERATE SON FRANKLIN MOORE

BORN JULY 10, 1846, DIED SEPTEMBER 18, 1864

He is on one knee staring at the headstone. Michelle walks up from behind and puts her hand on his shoulder.

Daniel ponders aloud, "He was 18. Am I the first person to look at this in over a hundred years?" He takes one of the flowers she's holding and puts one on his grave.

Hours later, from an open window, Michelle is helping Daniel undress his tie from behind as he stands in front of a dresser mirror. She's dressed tightly in black from the funeral in such a way that enhances her feminine beauty. He notices her for the first time since she arrived. Her soft black hair, waving just past her shoulders. Her wedding hand gently touches his cheek as her emerald eyes search into his. He's always loved her painted long nails. Her attractiveness seems ageless to him. His heightened senses return as he hears her breath into his ear.

Softly, "You understand, I have to leave tonight?"

She turns off the lamp and the last of the natural light is shaping her curves. She starts pulling out his shirt and unbuttoning it from the top. Successful, she then rubs her hands on his chest.

"Yes. I understand," he's becoming intoxicated by her innuendo.

She starts undoing his belt. He's watching her hands with intent.

"The cab's not for a couple hours," she moves with sheer seduction.

He now places his hands behind her on her buttocks. She starts breathing heavier. She takes one hand and pulls down her blouse and reveals her bra to tease him further. She guides one of his hands to her soft face.

Daniel is breathing heavy, "Michelle, I ..."

She turns toward him as her skirt falls to the floor and she starts pulling him to the bed.

"Not now," she quiets his objections, "Just take me."

He embraces her lips and slowly lays her down, falling into the moistness of her lips.

"Ah. Ah," Michele is now moaning.

Daniel is breathing heavier, "You feel so good."

"How I've missed you," Michelle says faintly

After a bit of time to reconnect, hearing the cab approach was bittersweet.

A few days later, it's a new morning, and the living room doorbell is ringing. Daniel opens the door in his sweat pants to greet Aunt Margret.

"I hope I'm not too early. I brought your mother's personal items and memorabilia she left for you. I figured I'd go through her storage, as painful as it was, it would've been much harder for you."

He looks on the porch and sees a few cardboard boxes and an antique metal box, a sword and a few kerosene lanterns. "You're right Margret, I couldn't have handled it. Thank you. And no, you're not too early. Come in."

He slides the items inside the door and into the foyer while she looks around and notices the large living room with a fireplace and mantle. There's contemporary furniture with a few paintings, vases, lamps and accessories, aesthetically balanced in every space.

"My, this looks lovely," Aunt Margret gushes. "You've done such a nice job in such little time."

Daniel proudly invites her in, "Come see the kitchen."

He walks her into the large kitchen still holding one plastic tub. It's bright with a large island and cooking area with a round breakfast table near a window viewing the back balcony and woods. It's laid out nicely around a marble island with state-of-the-art kitchen utensils and hanging lights.

"Oh, your mother would've been so impressed. She told me you wanted this… for her to stay here." She relieves a tear with her handkerchief. He then sets the box on the table and pulls out a leather binder with a feather quill attached. He gently puts his hand on her shoulder.

"Thank you. Have a seat. Let's have some tea."

She sits and looks at the binder.

"That sounds perfect," she agrees. "Why, that's his writing pen and paper." She peers over and pulls out a photograph. He brings two cups with some natural honey and a white ceramic pot on a tray, then sets it on the table.

Daniel observing, "Here you go, Margret."

"Oh, I haven't seen this since I was little. Daddy kept all this in a closet in the basement. We used to sneak down there and get into everything."

Daniel gently picks up the photograph tintype. "This is?" The photograph reveals a Union military portrait of a young handsome male in uniform.

"James A. Montgomery. Your great-great grandfather. He died at Andersonville Prison."

Daniel sets it down.

"That must be his sword, the one I handled when I was a boy."

She rummages through a few more photos. "Yes, he was a Sergeant in the Union Army, and there should be his letters to his wife somewhere in here, too. His handwriting was so eloquent."

Daniel glances over the items, then moves near the window looking out as if not being able to stay connected.

Aunt Margret noticing, asked, "You prefer to be alone?" She pauses. "Forgive me if I just like to retrospect".

"That's fine," he responds solemnly.

"She loved our family history, but got so detained by your father's prolonged illness that she never got to piece it all together."

"Life has a way of making detours." He looks out beyond the creek into the layers of trees. Misty clouds are moving in slightly, fogging the wooded view.

"The family legend has it that before Andersonville, he had escaped another prison the year before. He managed to make it all the way home to Missouri on furlough, where he spent one night with his wife. He told her if he ever got captured again he might not survive. Well, that one night they were together, she conceived. He rejoined his regiment in Mississippi, from where he wrote to her faithfully. In one of his letters, he speaks of a coming child with such anticipation. But, he was captured while out on a detail shortly after. He died within four months, in 1864, from the horrid conditions at Andersonville Prison."

Daniel turns and toasts his tea cup, breaking a slight smile "Here's to that one night."

She agrees in response and sips quietly.

"There's one problem. The timing and story was a bit too narrow for some. His older brother lived in the same town and was at home during the war. Some say he fathered the child."

Daniel disturbed, "Who says?"

"Those Baptist cousins of yours," she says a bit snarky, "The ones at the funeral. Guess they're still bitter being Southerners and all. Never the less, it bothered your mother greatly. She was determined to get to the truth."

He's more curious now, "So, what did they say on his wife's side? Her family?"

She looks puzzled. "I have no idea. Her letters are missing. I don't know anything about her side."

THUNDER cracks a short distance.

"Oh my. These storms can move in fast. I need to get going."

"Thanks for coming by. It was comforting."

She moves toward him and holds him in a warm embrace. "I'm always here." She withdraws and takes a long look at him. "How's your heart doing?"

"Jittery, but better."

More THUNDER sounds.

"Gotta go!" she said with urgency.

Daniel sees her to the door and watches her drive off. He looks at the items she has left in his possession and retires to his room, leaving them for another time. It begins to rain.

Daniel is lying in bed that evening and puts down a book as he drifts into sleep. A short time passes. He awakens to turn out the light when strangely it goes off and on again a few times on its own. The weather is quiet. His window is open to the dark of night outside. Within a few seconds he hears noises coming from the back yard, getting more pronounced. He turns the light back on, peeks out the window, and catches an owl hooting.

Daniel shouts at the owl, as if screeching at each other, "You're keeping me up."

The Letter

Another morning, afternoon, and evening go by without Daniel leaving his bed. Before sleep, he goes down to the kitchen and pours a glass of wine and selects a few crackers to go with it. He notices the tub and decides to carry it upstairs to the bedroom. He sits on the edge of his bed, grabs a letter and puts on a pair of reading glasses. *Fascinating.*

January 1864.

My Dearest, Most Affectionate wife, I am taking this time with pen hoping that these few words will find you in good health and great blessing. Today is the first day that I have been able to take my eyes off your last letter only because a fresh one has just arrived, the first in several weeks. My heart cannot go but a day without hearing your voice in verse on these pages. When you speak of such fondness of birds and Nightingales and compare our love to the force of nature, I can't help but share these rhythmic and beautiful themes with my fellow soldiers in camp. Please forgive me but I am so proud of your skill with poetic language and they have not heard from their loved ones for some time. Some for months. Their hearts are worn, as well they should be in this detestable war, yet when I read to them they forget where they are. So please write more often. I do not blame you for I understand the mail has been getting interrupted. My dearest Rachel, it is with great sorrow that I must inform you that my younger brother Jonah, who adored you so, and I know that you cared much for him, has lost his life in a battle with typhoid. I shall not burden you further with my heavy loss as you well know my care for him. His commander said he was a brave and wonderful soldier to have served under him. Could you tend to his wife Anna with letter as I will do also. She must be in the pangs of sorrow and weary with grief. I am making this short as I just mailed you seven pages yesterday. Your true and affectionate husband, James A. Montgomery.

Daniel whispers to himself "Wow, what heart...such an open soul."

He grabs another document and reads a short timeline of history. He looks at the date on the letter, then back to the document.

"My God, he'd be dead in a few months!"

He downs the wine and lies back down. He sees a photograph peeking out of a book. He pulls it out. It's his young mother with him as a child. He loses it. The sounds of a man sobbing drift outside into the night, then the light goes out. Shuffling noises among the crisp leaves continue as an occasional calling of a night owl echoes from the distance.

The following morning, the warmth of a new day's sun beams down on the deck. Daniel's hand is trying to imitate cursive writing from the letter of his ancestor while seated at a white wicker chair and table. Laid out in front of him are newly purchased art materials, a calligraphy set, a suede leather journal, and a large flashlight near a glass of wine by the bottle from which it was poured. He's focused on the penmanship. The breeze blows by twirling and shimmering the leaves, now his favorite visual and background noise.

"Hello?" from a short distance, the sound of Miss Fitzgerald's voice is carried across the acreage.

Daniel looks up from his interrupted concentration. She's below, walking around from the front, carrying flowers.

"I'm on the deck."

She steps up, well dressed, in sunglasses and hat.

Daniel politely surprised, greets her, "Hello...Sheila."

"I tried the front door. These are for you, Mr. Daniel, sir. My deepest sympathy." She points toward the kitchen door. "May I?"

He nods. She brings out a pitcher of water and arranges the flowers beautifully near him. He sees her iPhone camera and gestures.

"Thank you. Please. Would you mind?" He puts on his sun glasses and has a feather quill pen in hand by the new colorful bouquet of flowers.

"What a painting," she flatters.

He poses. She snaps, and then shows him.

Amused, "I want to show my agent. Let him know my next manuscript, if ever, will be hand-written."

"Well, I should let you be alone. You're working on your next novel."

Sincerely insisting, "No, please, stay."

She sits next to him, facing the forest.

"Hardly my next novel. He thinks I'm halfway through and I haven't even a story. Normally, I have a dozen in my head trying to decide which one to start. They're all meaningless now. Someone else can have them. Look."

He shows her his calligraphy sample. And, childlike, asks, "What do you think?"

"How lovely."

He holds up his journal.

"No more lap tops, cell phones, technology. I have no more to say or give to the world. This journal, my pen, and a glass of wine, this is my canvas now. Would you care for a glass?" he asks, mocking his gift of writing.

"Oh, no thank you. I envy your way with words Mr. Daniel. Please, never stop sharing your gifts and talents with us. The world needs people like you, and time will nurse back that romantic in you."

"This balcony is my world now. These trees are my friends."

"Well, perhaps they have a story to tell. We're like them in a way, going through the seasons of our lives."

He smiles, then imitates her Southern drawl. "Why Miss Fitzgerald. I do believe you have a flare of the romantic in you. And might I say, you are looking in the springtime of your life."

She laughs blushingly. "Why, Mr. Daniel sir, I do believe I'll have that glass of wine now," exaggerating her accent.

He pours her a glass and they both lean back watching a light gust flow through the chattering leaves. A flock of honking geese pass swiftly, flying low overhead, beyond the tops of the trees.

Daniel looking up pauses to ask, "Do you believe in signs?"

While grinning impishly, "I suppose, if they were flying over L.A. I would. But here, they're getting ready for the change to come."

Contemplating her answer, he agrees, "Yes, migration, driven by an invisible force. Fascinating."

The air current picks up and bends the trees slightly swaying back and forth. The pages of Daniel's empty journal start turning.

In the late-night quiet of his bedroom, the lights are flickering and suddenly go out. Noises from outside sound more human now. Daniel gets up slightly frightened, and grabs his new flashlight. He shines it outside his window into the back, then decides to light a kerosene lantern and put it on his dresser. He reaches into his cabinet and pulls out a fifth of Jack Daniels, pours it into a small glass and downs it. He crawls back under the covers. He's never felt so alone and scared.

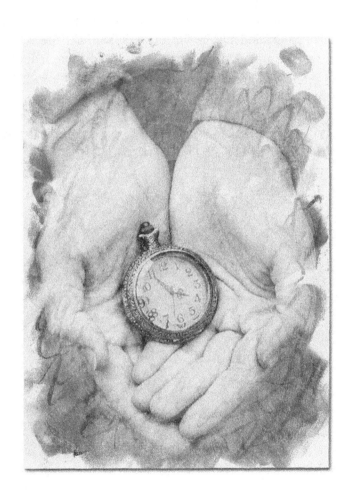

Somewhere in Time

Daniel's finishing his morning shower routine. He walks into the kitchen looking fresh and awake, wearing his full-length robe. The sunshine is breaking through. He pours his usual cup of coffee and opens the doorway out onto the balcony, then steps outside. He looks out as he is about to take a sip and freezes like a deer in the headlights. His eyes widen and his face has an expression of astonishment. He's startled by the panoramic view in front of his eyes.

PANNING BACK AND FORTH, ALMOST ENCIRCLING HIM, REVEALS THE ENTIRE BACK ACREAGE ACROSS THE CREEK IS ENCAMPED BY HUNDREDS OF CONFEDERATE SOLDIERS.

Most are dressed in uniform, but some are not. There are layers of smoldering campfires among the dozens of tents. Many horses are neighing, exhaling the cold air. Some men are cooking, others washing clothes by the creek, even one is bathing in a heated tub. Many lay sleeping on the ground under wool blankets. Others are cleaning rifles, while some are tending wounded.

The breeze picks up, blowing those same leaves, but a different setting below. Daniel sets down his coffee without taking his eyes off the scene beneath. Suddenly, a flock of honking geese fly overhead, forcing Daniel to look up and catch the identical formation from the previous day vanish into an invisible line in the sky as if into another dimension.

He scurries downstairs and steps out onto the ground. He pauses and looks left to right, confused by the change of scenery. He contemplates another shot of whiskey, but keeping clear-headed, steps into the back acreage of his yard and walks toward the creek then stands at the bank. He spots three young boys gathered around a smoldering fire.

"What are you doing here?" he calls out, squinting if perhaps it was an illusion.

They offer no answer. From the creek's edge, he stretches one leg toward them, stepping on one rock, and then reaches the bank on the other side. His robe turns to a long wool coat in a mystical moment. He begins to walk through the tent area with trepidation. The men are going about their business, acknowledging him, but giving little concern. He walks with a bit more trust then approaches and stops by one soldier, a young boy, stooping and cooking with a pan over a fire.

"Is this some sort of reenactment?"

The boy glances up at him, but gives no response. He asks the other soldier, "How old are you?"

One boy stands and spits, eyeing him up and down.

"Seventeen, sir."

Daniel, feigning a grin, and sensing relief exclaims, "You're a Scout troop, right?"

The third boy sharpens his knife, but says nothing.

"Learning survival skills. That's good," Daniel juxtapositions a more cautious tone.

Daniel again tries to uncover this strange scene. "Seriously, what are you doing here?"

The one boy seems more talkative, with a strong country Southern twang; he is the first to explain, "Texas Brigade, sir. We're holding Sandy Creek til further orders."

"You're holding my back yard!" Daniel exclaims.

They all look at him.

Quickly, cautious again, Daniel covers up his remarks, "That's good," as he looks around suspiciously. "Holding it from who?"

"Yankees! Maybe two days out. Got us on the run fer now. Waiting orders from General Hood where to ambush 'em."

The third one, sharpening his knife, chimes in barely understandable, "That yorn house yonder? Yuz got any chikns?"

Daniel turns back and sees his house, then looks back to the soldier with a crazy expression. "Yorn? You guys are good. Really, what's going on?" It's all incredulous to him.

The Rebel boy cooking holds out a frying pan after taking a sample. "Take ye' some. Darn tasty beins brown tail."

Daniel looks about questioning as his thoughts trying to rationalize what his eyes are seeing and his ears are hearing. The friendlier rebel boy spits again. "Squirrel meat," he pauses. "You ain't got nothin ta worry about, sir. We won't bother yer house."

Daniel decides to look around more. He pets a horse on the face, then glances further. He notices two officers looking over a map outside a tent with a table so he then walks toward them. They stand straight and look his way.

The first uniformed officer looks up and notices a some-what nervous Daniel approaching. With an educated tone of comfort, he assures him "We won't be needing your house, if that's what you're seeking."

"Well, that's a relief."

He looks at the map with puzzlement. "You're lost, right?"

"No sir. This is Sandy Creek Ridge, yonder is Sugar Hill. Cavalry scouted the area a fortnight back."

The other officer looks over Daniel then, with a deep good ol' boy voice, "You seen any Yanks?"

Quickly, a civilian rider pulls up and slides off his horse with a saddle bag full of mail. He dumps it out on the table and then hands the officers specially tied letters.

The rider is out of breath, "Ya'lls lucky I got through. Yanks everywhere twixt here and Atlanta. No more mail lieutenant, this is it."

They quickly hand him some water and food while he then hops back on his horse and rides off. Daniel's mouth is open.

The second officer grimaces, "That settles it."

They go back to their map.

"Agreed. Hood ain't comin. We'll retreat further south."

Daniel walks around unnoticed to where he can see the mail. He picks up an envelope and reads the postmark. AUGUST 19, 1864

He then picks up a post card, dated the same year, with perfect cursive handwriting.

My dearest beloved husband, the war can wait. Our children are hungry and crying for their father. Please come home. Your devoted wife, Martha May.

Daniel sets it down in awe, completely perplexed. "Excuse me. This is dated August 1864. These letters are all dated…"

They chuckle and look at each other grinning "That's only a month late. Least it's the same year." More laughter. Now Daniel looks around in disbelief. He makes one last attempt at clarity.

"In that case, could I borrow your telephone? Mine's dead."

They look at him with blank stares and dead silence.

Daniel politely dismisses his request, "Never mind then."

He looks at his wrist, but there's no watch. "It seems I've lost track of time."

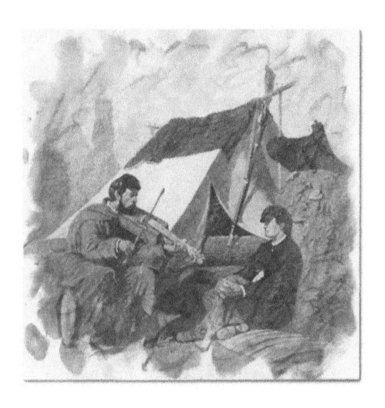

A Rebel Soldier's Dying Wish

Later that night in his bedroom, Daniel begins his journal:

*It sorrows me deeply, that on the first page of my
journal, is written with such a troubled heart, that
I believe that the pen I now hold, is in the hand of
a man gone insane.*

Daniel looks out his open window and sees campfires.
He's wearing a full-length coat with scarf and his breath is
fogging in the crisp air as he picks up the land line and dials,
listening to the recorded voice on the other end.

Female voice: "The time and date is now 12:09 AM,
Wednesday, September 18th. Current temperature is 43
degrees as a cold front is moving through. Today's high
will be 49 ...".

Click. He hangs up, grabs a fifth of Jack Daniels, his
mother's cigarettes, a map, and heads outside. As he does,
the power goes out again.

He steps through the creek water and up to a campsite
outside what appears to be an infirmary tent. It's cold. He
sets down by three young soldiers that are awake among
the many who are asleep under their blankets. He passes

out cigarettes and offers whiskey around the campfire. They gladly accept and hold out cups and light up. There's an older, bearded one who is tuning his rustic fiddle. The younger one is shaking and fumbling inside his coat, so Daniel moves closer by his side and wraps a blanket around him. He coughs with a deep chest rattle.

The weak, young one asks of Daniel, "Could you help me? I want to see my letter by the fire."

Daniel reaches and pulls out a letter and the envelop slips to the ground. He hears the sound of the fiddle turn to a soft but raw violin solo.

"I'd be obliged if you would read it to me, sir…my mother and my darling fiancé."

Daniel notices some yellowing and frayed edges that indicate it's an old letter. He looks over at the other soldier who sort of shakes his head at the sad affair.

Daniel takes a swig, squats down, then clears his throat, "*Dearest son, I hope this letter reaches you the way I remember you, so loving and full of mischief. I miss you so and find all* my *prayers lay with hopes and dreams of your safe return. Your things are just as you left them, with an extra pair of socks and shirt I have sewn from a dress I need no longer wear.*"

The boy coughs and Daniel gives him a swig. He's struggling to stay upright.

"Could you skip to the part about my Molly?"

He looks over as the weakened soldier is leaning so he sits by him as to hold him up. The campfire reflects his eyes and youthful face.

The music continues to drift through the campsite.

Daniel finds the written few words, "*Sweet Molly, your young wife-to-be, has come by and left some flower petals to send with this letter. Her brother's absence keeps her busy on the farm but she promises to write when she can.*

She says to tell you her heart will always be yours. Come home soon from this dreaded war son, and we'll be waiting for you. Your loving mother, Emily Moore."

Weaker now, he softly says, "Thank you so kindly," he drifts off. "I will close my eyes...and go to her".

Daniel now sees that he's dying. Holding him, he picks up the fallen envelope with his free hand. It reads:

PVT. FRANKLIN MOORE

He looks with a stare of astonishment. *This can't be happening.*

He holds the boy through the long night. He dies in his arms.

Morning comes without sleep. Daniel watches from a short distance as they put him into a shallow grave with a rock pile then he turns and walks away.

At the headquarter tent, an officer is drinking coffee at the table. Daniel pulls out the map and sets it out in front of them.

"Your maps are a little out dated." He hesitates to offer more advice, then asks, "May I have the boy's things? I'll make sure they get to his mother, she'll want to bury him properly."

The officer nods affirmative.

Daniel continues in his journal:

> *I was saddened after long hours with one young 18-year-old boy, coughing and cold, away from home, who pulled out a treasured letter from his mother and asked if I would read it to him. It was dated over a year old, 1863. Yet his heart was with his beloved Molly and he drifted into the night to be with her, never to awaken again. I could detect tear drops on the ink from times read before. As he*

lay there, his name jumped out at me from his grave.
Franklin Moore. It was him, from the gravestone at
my mother's funeral, and today was the exact date
on the granite marker. I was overwhelmed with a
feeling of utter helplessness. I looked at his pic-
ture of Molly when I returned and wept. I held him
through the night until his last breath at dawn. They
took him away for burial. I kept his belongings and
vowed, somehow, to contact his mother.

Daniel takes a drink then stands and looks out the
window at the back acreage...

Which begs the question.

... as the cold wind blows and the distant trees bend and
sway above the pile of rocks marking Franklin Moore's
lonesome grave.

Why is the fate of this lad's final place of rest in the
hands of a mortal writer lost in time?

Daniel hears the mail vehicle out front then dashes outside to catch him. He comes running out in his robe waving
to Henry by the mail box, a distance at the end of a long
driveway. The vehicle starts to pull away then stops.

Daniel out of breath is able to spurt out, "Please. I
need a favor."

At the back acreage, Henry comes around the house
with Daniel toward the creek as Daniel stops.

"Tell me...Henry. What do you see?"

Henry views an empty forest across the creek with a
sloping hill above a valley to the right.

"A winding creek... a forest...few birds."

Daniel is staring across the creek. The Confederate
encampment is still present to his sight.

Henry can make none of it out, only he's now starting
to show concern for Daniel.

"You're sure? No people? Can you hear anything?" Daniel implores the post man.

He looks farther left, then right, then back at Daniel.

Henry hesitates, but admits, "No. Nothing. Are you all right Mr. Coffee?"

Daniel falls to a seated position with his head in his hands in desperate frustration. A hawk soars above, higher and higher. Below, a vast view of two worlds, in separate time, clearly visible to this man who once stumbled upon a grave marker and wondered aloud, and now, was stuck in a time portal, between two worlds.

A Question Of Sanity

Daniel is seated across from a female psychiatrist in her 40's. She was one of the numbers the nurse handed to him for grief counseling. He's clean shaven, well dressed, and styled his hair with gel as if he's giving an interview for a position he desperately needs. She is rather stoic, while Daniel fidgets, then makes known her assessment after taking some notes.

"Your experience is quite troubling. Even bizarre, however..."

"Do you believe me?"

She changes position. "It's not a matter whether I believe you or not, Mr. Coffee, it's certainly real to you. Perhaps your sub-conscious is acting something out. You have no history of hallucinating disorders, drugs, seizures, it's obviously attributable to the trauma of your mother's sudden death. Then add the stress from your career, and a marriage on the rocks."

Daniel defensively corrects her, "I said I wasn't sure about my marriage."

"In any event...let's call it Acute Trauma Disorientation. You first experienced it in the hospital when you said every-thing was spinning."

Daniel's body language is increasingly discomforting.

"Yes, but this is not spinning. This is real."

She sighs. "But not real to your mailman. Let's at least get a handle on your physical health, like sleep, eating... and slow down on the drinking. Meantime, this should help you relax."

She writes out a prescription and hands it to him.

Daniel drives up to his house and sees a very tall black man wearing sunglasses, walking two dogs, with a shapely female by his side. It's J.J. Bynum. They're dressed in designer sweats and stand out with a lot of bling. Daniel stops at the driveway entry to check his mail when J.J. approaches.

"Name's J.J., w'sup neighbor? I live across the way," pointing to his house and being genuinely friendly.

Daniel holds out his hand, a bit spooked by the dogs. They shake hands. "Daniel."

J.J. looks Daniel's car over.

"Like your ride. Old school," J.J. says with a cool tone. "Say, we been havin' some parties, just come on up whenever you feel like. Plenty a booze and some fine ladies."

Daniel glances at his woman, then the dogs while she gives him a cute once over and makes him feel a little uneasy.

"Sure, might take you up on that," Daniel says.

J.J.'s cell rings when one dog seems to yelp at Daniel.

Daniel remarks to her, "Will there be a lot of dogs there? We don't get along too well."

"Come as you are, handsome, the girls don't bite," she answers rather amused.

J.J. on the phone starts another conversation, "Yo. Wussup?"

He nods at Daniel, then they walk away.

Inside the kitchen his land line phone rings. Daniel sees the caller ID is Jason but he picks up the phone reluctantly. "Aright, so, how'd you get my number?"

"Your wife called me, she's concerned about you."

"Yeah…" Daniel sees troop movement through the window and is now distracted.

"Yeah, quite frankly, so am I. She said you sounded incoherent last time she called. That's tragic about your mom, but…"

Daniel has a strange look on his face when he opens the door and lowers the phone.

"… you gotta keep it together." Jason snaps.

Daniel is greatly distracted outside. The time portal has crossed the creek halfway up to his house with a trail parallel to his creek. He lifts the phone back to his ear.

"I gotta go," Click.

He stands outside at the trail across the way and sees all the Confederate soldiers clearing out. The same officer he spoke with is mounting a horse. Daniel can hear a THUNDEROUS RUMBLE in the far distance, then the officer addresses Daniel from across the creek.

"Yanks bout a day's ride from here. Hood says we got to meet up further West and we're outta supplies. Might want to take flight yourself… they'll ravage your goods. Civilians are fleeing Atlanta. That's the shelling you hear, they say it's like hail on fire. God almighty himself has abandoned Dixie!" He tips his hat and trots South West.

Daniel watches. "Yanks," He is laughing. "Yanks!"

He now starts looking up and turning in circles shouting, "The Yankees are coming!" Laughing hysterically. From up and away Daniel is spinning a bit madly, holding his arms out, trying to stable his universe.

The Quantum Equation

T he crowded, fast moving pace of downtown Atlanta contrasts sharply with the rural setting of Summerville. The following late morning, Daniel walks into a doorway carrying a brief case and the civil war sword with a piece of scratch paper looking around for a directory. He sees the history exhibit on the second floor but accidently hits the third-floor button in the elevator. He steps out and looks both ways. As he walks by an open doorway, sounds of electricity, radio frequencies and bubbles fill the large room full of tubes, colored flashing lights, and a white Persian cat napping on top a high stack of books.

Daniel curious, carefully calls out, "Hello?'

POOF. A puff of smoke rises from behind a strange machine startling Daniel. A slight built Asian man with hair going several directions emerges wearing a white lab coat, an eye protective shield and heavy gloves. He lifts his eye wear.

His broken dialect expresses his frustration "Wrong wave length. Need less pressure".

"Pressure?" Daniel asks.

He pulls out a large roast duck, well over-cooked, smoking with a concoction of noodles. "My invention. Cooks duck Chow Mein in 30 seconds. Anything, chicken, steak, pork...30 seconds. This time too much. OK, taste it."

Daniel rolls with it. "Sure, squirrel for breakfast, duck for dinner." He takes a bite with the utensil he hands him as the quirky character watches Daniel with anticipation. Mouth swirling, "That's delicious for being overdone...Mr....?"

"Emo. Professor Emo. You from the government about the solar flare? The map is there on the wall and I'll print out the data if you like."

Daniel turns and sees a large wall map with pins and lights of different color. He walks closer and looks it over with fascination.

"I wish I was government, Professor Emo, that would simplify my life right now. I'm just Daniel. I actually came to find the history museum and curator. What does all this mean?"

Professor Emo removes the gloves and eye wear and pridefully explains.

"These are control, directly linked with NASA. A hot line was set up to report all incoming incidents possibly related to unusual solar activity. It's every kind of story from paranormal to just plane bizarre."

Daniel tunes in. "How bizarre? You mean like crazy?"

"Oh, no, Mr. Daniel, nothing is crazy to me. I am lead investigative scientist of The Source Field Project, dedicated to all energy that's measurable and how it affects our universe and planet - my Quantum Equation. Just because it is unusual or unseen doesn't make it crazy."

Daniel's interest is now peaking. "Ok, give me an example."

Emo looks up, finds his laser pointer and points.

"Yes. Here in Japan, ships in harbor are gone... missing."

Daniel, not easily akin to the abnormal, is now open. "Just like that?"

Emo points elsewhere. "Just like that. Here, children in school gym floating in the air with no explanation."

"What?" he is amazed.

The excitable professor points again, now he's found a listener. "Rancher and 200 head of cattle in Wyoming discovered one hour later in soccer stadium in Portugal."

Daniel is making faces. "And you don't think that's crazy?"

Emo looks at Daniel with an exaggerated, wise and confident smile.

"I am Professor Emo, MIT graduate, top of my class all time. Over 100 patents and 1000 pending. I have written several books and Nobel Prize winner twice, would have been three times but my theory was too far over their heads." He walks Daniel over to several mechanical devises that are unrecognizable. "The reason it is not crazy to me is because I can explain these once I examine the facts. Whether they believe me, that's another matter. NASA pays me big money, I make my inventions, and conduct experiments, give them the study and findings, then they file everything away top secret."

Daniel is now eager to further explore. "So, explain say… the floating children."

"One word Mr. Daniel. Energy. Altered states of energy, all interconnected by the invisible Source Field."

Daniel questions him to explain, "OK, OK, so, the floating, energy, no gravity, you're saying the sun flares are causing that? How?"

Emo writes on the board. "Pulsation, plus location, plus magnetic field, divided by time, will give you your answer. The Quantum Equation."

Daniel is figuring in his mind.

Professor Emo continues, "The gym was built on a vortex, according to my grid. These vortices are worldwide and produce a ranging magnetic field that can pull or create opposing energy to counter balance the field. In this case, in a moment of time, the gravity was neutralized at the exact moment children were traumatized and triggered the perfect effect of floating in air."

Daniel catches a phrase, "Wait, the children triggered it?"

Emo adds one more equation on the board to the previous. "My bad; in some cases, you must add the human element. The heart has an electromagnetic field that projects eight feet out from our bodies. Any sudden trauma can affect its vibration frequency, sometimes to such an extreme as to alter the balance of the Source Field. Ironically, a child tragically fell from the stands right in front of all of them. That triggered the collective heart field at the same time the solar pulse had hit the vortex. Bingo. That is why it is not crazy to me."

Daniel points to his formula. "OK. That's fascinating, what about the ships? The sun is the pulse, then the flares provide a blast of energy rippling through space."

Laser points to time factor. "Rippling through space and time, Mr. Daniel - it alters space and time."

Daniel's eyes get big. "Whoa, alter time? Now you've got my absolute attention."

Emo continues, "The ships are still there, they just can't see them or detect them. Unless you were on the same frequency..."

"Then you could see them?" Daniels asks hopefully.

Emo is flattered. "You are learning my son," he says tongue and cheek. "Of course, without the original cause, the solar flares, none of this would be happening."

"How are you sure the ships are still there?"

"Good question Mr. Daniel. My assistant took instruments to measure the field readings. They are there."

Daniel is now intrigued. He hesitates but poses the question. "Could you measure readings from my house? My property?"

Emo looks at him detached, as his thoughts are wandering back to his cooking formula.

"Maybe alternate angle for wave length," Emo ponders.

Daniel tries again. "I'll pay you, I need your help."

Emo now assesses Daniel's concern. Probably a low-level situation, similar to others he's often asked to remedy.

"Mr. Daniel, my assistant has all our equipment and is currently overseas on assignment."

Daniel looks disappointed then sighs and recites a quote

"My grief lies all within, and these external matters
of lament, are merely shadows of the unseen grief,
that swells with silence in the tortured soul."

He pauses. "For a second I thought I was led here by a better fate than what has befallen my mind and heart."

Emo cocks his head. "Nobody talks that way. You have something peculiar going on. I am suspect. I have seen that look in other clients. Give me your address and I might investigate the matter."

Daniel writes it down, then says, "Shakespeare."

"Excuse me?" Emo quizzes.

"William Shakespeare. He talked that way 400 years ago. Where can I find, um..." looking at scratch paper, "Professor Langley?"

Emo frowns. "That nut job! He's a Harvard grad. He's so full of himself. Second floor history museum by the Civil War exhibit. Such a fool that man. Make fun of my work."

Emo puts his gloves and eye wear on, mumbling under his breath, while he grabs another duck and starts up the machine. The cat jumps from its perch to hide, meanwhile Daniel has a new bounce in his step. It's OK to be crazy.

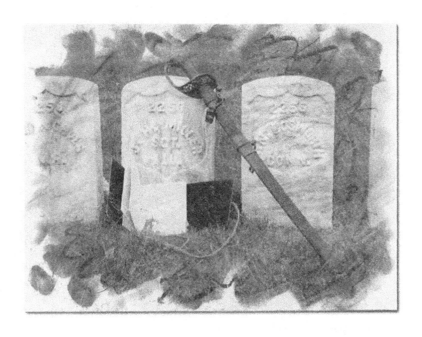

Andersonville

On the second floor of the science building, Daniel is engrossed at the wall of the Cyclorama battle collage, a 360-degree infamous oil painting depicting a myriad of scenes at The Battle of Atlanta, during the Civil War.

A male voice assumes to narrate from behind the massive, panoramic mural, "The famous Hurt House and the Battle for Atlanta. This battle cost several thousand lives, which could have been avoided but Southern politicians were such fools - Jeff Davis chief among them."

Daniel turns to see a slightly older gentleman, short in stature, with head full of silvering, wavy hair and a scholarly beard. He reaches out his hand. "Professor Langley, my students and colleagues call me Brandy, after General Sherman's favorite drink."

Daniel changes arms holding the sword and shakes his hand. "I'm Daniel. Daniel Coffee, I like it with or without Brandy." They chuckle. "In fact, I was given your name from a librarian. I'd like to authenticate, or at least get some background on who my ancestor was, the owner of this sword."

Brandy glances at his sword and holds out his hand as Daniel hands it to him.

"It's actually referred to as a saber," he clarifies. "Step into my office."

Inside his office are walls of books, Civil War memorabilia, photographs of Lincoln, Grant, Lee, Sherman, and several framed photographs of Brandy participating in Union uniform during battle reenactments. On his desk are an open leather scrapbook and a magnifying glass on top.

"I was just finishing my telegram collection. Rare telegrams – well, outside of the Smithsonian. They were used to exchange communications between Grant, Sherman and President Lincoln."

"And you authenticate them how?" Daniel inquires.

Brandy grabs a thick book from the shelf. "I'm old school, it's rare when I use a computer. This volume details every telegram on record which I've come to memorize with great detail."

He opens for Daniel to glance. "Maps, oh yes, and maps..." he pulls out another volume "...without those topographers, they'd been running around in circles."

Again, Daniel observes and is a bit fascinated at what passion this man has for history.

"At the beginning of the war the maps were as outdated as that saber is today."

"You might be surprised." Daniel remarks from his first-hand encounter.

Brandy sets the saber down on the desk and pulls it out of its leather sheath.

"I tried cleaning the rust off," Daniel adds.

Brandy looks closer. "That's not rust, that's blood stains. Are you a history buff, Mr. Coffee?"

"Fiction. Except for art and literature, I've never had much interest in the past - until now."

Daniel takes out several letters and puts them in front of Brandy. He then puts on his spectacles. "Let's see what we have."

Daniel gets to the real point of his search, "What do you know about Andersonville?"

Brandy stops his thumbing through letters and looks at Daniel over his spectacles.

"Andersonville was the worst prison in American history; an epitaph of man's utter inhumanity to man. If Sherman would've marched to the walls of that abyss before his famous campaign to the sea, Georgia would never have survived the wrath and slaughter of an Army gone mad."

He pulls out a picture of what appears to be a Holocaust survivor. Daniel gasps.

"Yes, here in America," he emphasizes pointedly.

He puts the photo away then proudly keeps talking, while continuing to examine the artifacts.

"I take my students there twice a year and I'm considered the leading expert in the country. My masters at Harvard..."

Daniel instantly insists, "Take me there."

Brandy looks at him over his spectacles again. Daniel pulls out from inside his sport coat the leather wallet from his ancestor. "I'll pay you whatever you want, my ancestor is buried there. Just tell your boss..."

Brandy stiffens, "I am Professor William T. Langley as in William Tecumseh Sherman and I call the shots here. This is my operation."

Daniel tugs on a few more bills to entice him further.

Smiling a bit arrogantly, "I'll grab the Brandy and cigars, you take care of the food and driving."

A short time later, they're rolling down a rural highway as Brandy continues his examining the historical significance of Daniel's possessions.

"These letters are priceless. Hmmm. Illinois 31st Regiment. Under Sherman and McPherson. James

A. Montgomery. Strong name. Your mother's side of the family?"

"Yes. She died before she could piece together his story. I write stories myself, so she passed it on to me. I'm clueless as where to start, but it was her dying wish."

"Wait, you're that writer! Daniel Coffee. Yeah, I've seen your book covers…kinda catchy. I just can't get into fiction…but I might now. I might fancy a good adventure, been getting too routine lately."

Daniel looks over at Brandy then back at the road as they drive by an old abandoned town.

"Like a venture back in time maybe? That'll rock your routine."

Daniel finds some Bluegrass on the radio. The scenery evolves into some deeper, rural backwoods with hanging moss, a Bayou quality of life where everyone seems to be living on their porch. They pass by run- down brick buildings and shanty towns reflecting where blacks and whites live in Southern poverty. Daniel's eye is drawn to abandoned farms and horses in fields that remind him of so many paintings. Every ancient looking cemetery they pass now gives him an eerie feeling. He looks over at Brandy shuffling through his artifacts.

"Can you authenticate the Franklin Moore letters if they are dated correctly?" Daniel asks, still haunted by the surreal event

Brandy puts on his spectacles then he studies and compares.

"Indeed, they are; stamps a dead giveaway. Ink, writing style. The details speak for themselves. Why would you question this?"

"Right now, I have a lot of questions."

What seems a short time later, but really was more than two hours, they arrive at the Andersonville Prison National

Park. They pull around a vast field of large monuments with two large wooden remains of the stockade. There's a long slope down to a creek bed, basically in the middle of nowhere. When they park and get out, Daniel takes in the attractive sweeping view for a brief moment, just before being made aware that he's standing in the middle of a nightmare from his ancestor's past.

Brandy points to a remain of the stockade and begins his guided tour. "It was originally built to hold 9,000 prisoners. In less than a year there were 36,000 starving, dying, souls inside those walls." He points to an area that was once a creek bed. "Only one waterway in - a creek from above. Well, that's fine. The soldiers knew better to drink up top, wash in the center and let human waste run-off at the bottom. Only thing they didn't know was the confederates were doin' the same on the outside. The prisoners were drinkin' the rebels' crap! They never had a chance. Average life in there was 3 to 4 months - a regular Holocaust. An oven would've been more humane. The creek turned into a swamp of human feces, sometimes they were waist deep into it."

They walk by a make-shift medical tent as a breeze relieves the slight heat from the fall sun. Daniel realizes there was no shelter or trees in the compound area. *How long could I survive this misery?*

Brandy goes on to describe the anatomy of agony, "Most painful, suffering, slow death...do you know what dysentery and full-blown diarrhea does to a body, Mr. Coffee? The bacteria swells your guts the size of a basketball. You shit blood and maggots, sometimes a gallon an hour, with agonizing pain, and the stench...especially in a confined area. Then the muscles contract and you just lie there dying in your own filth, with worms crawling inside. There were up to 5,000 men in medical at any given time, with only two attendants. Word was if you made it to medical, you were a dead man."

Daniel is horrified. "This is a dark secret I never imagined."

Brandy points to two white sticks going all around the parameter.

"Between those outer and inner sticks was the deadline. Cross it and they shot you dead from those towers. The lucky ones were killed without the suffering."

Shortly after, they came walking out of the information center with a paper, a map, and a couple of books. Brandy is looking closer at a particular paper, designating the burial plot.

"James A. Montgomery is buried in section K."

They arrive at the sprawling, endless cemetery, and drive near the appropriate site. Getting out, Daniel is struck by the sea of granite grave stones laid out precisely and evenly in rows. He locates the one marked 4514 - James A. Montgomery, with his rank and regiment engraved. Daniel kneels down, and solemnly he vows, "I'm going to give you a voice. You deserve that much."

Brandy pauses in silence. He then takes the occasion to pull out a cigar from his pocket case and lights it with one puff. With some relief, he exhales and resumes his historical details.

"They carried out 100 bodies a day. Over 13,000 men are buried here. You see, they didn't plan to keep them, they were counting on the prisoner exchange continuing as usual. There was only one slight problem…"

Daniel looks to him for the answer as a black couple walk nearby. More tourists are relaxing on a concrete bench so they find one empty bench and Brandy sits down with Daniel.

"...the Negroes. They were now in uniform fighting alongside the Union, thanks to Lincoln and the Emancipation Proclamation. They fought well and proud - too well. When it came time for the customary exchanging of prisoners, the South wouldn't allow what few Negroes who were captive to go also. Georgia still considered them their property."

"Property?" Daniel repeats naively.

Brandy nods. "Lincoln and Grant were outraged."

Daniel looks at a black family getting out of a car. "So my great, great grandfather died because black Americans were thought of as property, not soldiers? My God, who ran this place?"

Brandy affirms, "I'll show you".

They enter the small town of Andersonville and walk the Main Street. They find a seat by a small, inconspicuous building marked Captain Wirz Headquarters.

Brandy continues, "Captain Henry Wirz. The only man to hang for war crimes after the Civil War ended. It was too much to forgive so they strung his ass up rather quickly."

They get up and take a walk. "If General Winder had lived long enough, he would've hanged too, as he was really the one who oversaw the Georgia prisons."

They walked a short distance and discovered a pre-served railroad depot with long tracks that seem to come from a distant nowhere, but it stands out as a major land-mark, as guilty as the prison itself.

"This must be how they came in," Daniel observes.

"Yep, their last stop ever. Then they marched themselves from here right to the gates of hell."

In the town museum, they walk through a gallery of photos, relics, diaries, and a handmade relief replica of the actual open field prison. On the wall reveals a photograph of the hanging of the warden, Captain Henry Wirz, in front of the Capital Building in Washington. Another startling photo reveals the ditches for graves of sorts - bodies being laid side-by-side, taken from a pile on top of a wagon. Another horrible graphic of a crowded stockade, men defecating over a makeshift bridge.

Daniel questions, "So many lives. Why didn't they escape?"

"They kept thinking there was going to be a prisoner exchange, and the rebels fueled that lie to keep 'em in the dark and so no riots. A few got out by tunneling. Most didn't make it."

Daniel continues looking at pictures, "So, knowing what you do, how would you have tried to escape?"

Brandy ponders a bit. "Outside of bribing a guard, I would fake my death. Let the trustees carry me to my grave like these." He points to the picture of the mass grave ditch.

"But how would you stay alive? How long would you have?"

"If I was going to die anyway, might as well be on my terms. A slim chance, but might have worked."

They walk into a nearby restaurant and bar and are seated near a few tourists, and some obvious Southern locals. Soon a waitress, carrying a bottle of brandy and two glasses, appears.

"Here you are, Professor Brandy, your favorite table and brandy for two."

Brandy puffed up a bit and added, "And my favorite waitress."

Daniel is impressed. There's a picture of General Sherman on the wall.

"Now there's a 'man's man, I portray him at re-enactments," Brandy brags.

He sticks the half-smoked cigar in his mouth and pours some brandy in a glass for both. He then stands and puts on a General's coat and hat from a dummy mannequin displaying a Union uniform, then puts his hand inside like in Sherman's famous picture where he is striking a pose.

Brandy with his head up, "What do ya think?"

Daniel is amused. "Hide the women and children."

Brandy takes it to the next level. "That's good". Loud in character, he proceeds to take the part seriously, "All right, you heard the man! Hide the women and children. William T. Sherman is givin' you one hour before we burn this village down...that is, if Maggie doesn't serve the best fried green tomatoes with her famous chili this side of Mason Dixon, then we're all goin' to hell."

He toasts Maggie, the chef, through her window and she waves him off and smiles. The crowd laughs as he sits down. Daniel's just witnessed a brilliant characterization.

"Such theater - you were made for this role."

Snickering, he replies, "So, you've heard the myth, he plundered and pillaged poor Georgia, burning down everything in sight. I have a theory, though. The South burned it down. The hatred for the Yankee was so vicious they would rather destroy Ole Dixie than see their Northern enemy have one ounce of Southern heritage." He leans down on the table and stares right into Daniels face with cynical sarcasm, "Especially let a 'Nigra' occupy the spoils,

God forbid!"

On the return trip, a couple of hours later, Daniel is driving and a slightly drunk Brandy is singing.

"When Johnny comes marching home again Hurrah! Hurrah! We'll give him a hearty welcome then, Hurrah! Hurrah!" Brandy was belting it out as Daniel drove.

Driving down the countryside road, Brandy can be heard outside the window with smoke billowing out. "Oh, the men will cheer, the boys will shout, the ladies they will all turn out. When Johnny comes marching home again..."

As evening closes in, Brandy gets out at his house and leans down to say good bye.

"Night my friend. Oh, by the way. That's not your ancestor's saber…"

"What do you mean?" Daniel is puzzled.

"It's an officer's saber of much higher rank. Sergeants didn't have those, that is, unless he wasn't just a Sergeant. Good night."

He salutes, leaving Daniel bewildered and with even more questions.

Looking for Answers

L ate the next morning, Daniel awakens and immediately looks out his window hoping for a 'back to reality'
moment. The worn pathway travelers have used runs by his
house but no one is visible except across the creek. He goes
downstairs and steps outside closer to the creek and feels
the fresh air as the last of the Confederates clear out. He
notices there is more moving about than normal. He thinks
about crossing further into the portal but hesitates. *I'll go
into town, grab a bite to eat, and then maybe break the news
to Michelle that I've gone mad.* His time with the two pro-
fessors was educational, but Daniel still needed answers.
Maybe they won't come from the world of science or history. *What alternatives do I have?*

Daniel pulls away from the Waffle House after eating
a late breakfast. He noticed Donna but she was way too
busy for a normal conversation. He decides to pay Aunt
Margret a visit and drives in the direction of her home.
Maybe talking with his Aunt would possibly ground him
back to center. He hoped so. He was willing to try anything
at this point.

Daniel remembered driving by, upon his original arrival,
what he was immediately amused with, especially in the
Bible belt of Georgia - a small, recently erected building,
with a sign that read Psychic Readings, surrounded by

colorful icons of Tarot cards, crystal balls and light bulbs shaped like stars.

Ironically, only a few hundred feet away was a large sign that read Church of Prophecy. That fact that this county would even allow a psychic was unusual, but how uncanny, competing with a church that specializes in future events in people's lives. What was once a visual amusement, now appealed to his search for answers. With Daniel's desperation and his keen sense from researching while writing novels, drove him to conquer the strange sequence of events, along with the pain of his mother's death,

His only experience with a medium prior was when he was a teen. He and a friend were walking around the Long Beach Pike, a small amusement park back in the day, frequented by sailors, dock workers, ports-au-call travelers and local retired folks. He remembers his friend daring him to go in with him to see the gypsy fortune teller. The typical hand painted attractive signs outside guaranteed your future fortunes and chances for romance. So, they went inside to a dark and mysterious atmosphere. Daniel immediately wanted to turn around, but she appeared quickly in gypsy garb and told them to be seated. Daniel left not remembering or relating to anything she said, but his friend seemed shaken and disturbed the rest of the evening.

What the hell, Daniel figures in his mind. He makes a U-turn and heads to the cite, hoping to find a glimmer of understanding. He chooses to pull into the small empty parking lot of the Clairvoyant first. The sign above the door reads 'Leave Your Preconceived Expectations and Skepticism at the Door.' He looks around inside and sees crystals, pyramid shaped objects and a sign with various prices.

"Welcome" a dainty white-haired woman in her early 60's steps out from behind a curtain.

"Hello, I'm new to this so…"

She points to the table "Please be seated." She reaches for his palms and turns them up. "You're a simple man with a complicated matter. I can do a simple reading or a spiritual guide, which would you prefer?'

"Oh no spirits, that's my problem. Are they real or…"

"Please, $20 then we'll proceed."

Daniel hands her a twenty "That seems reasonable."

"I'm Lydia," she smiles.

'Daniel,"

"Daniel, I sense no spirits at all. Why do you say they're a problem?"

"Not spirits. Well, you just clarified that matter. You're sure?"

"Yes. You are among the living. Many of them. So, I'll do personal item reading. Give me your ring please." He hands her his wedding ring. "It's warm with a vision," she senses.

"Well yes, my hands are warm. What vision?"

She puts the ring on a crystal and closes her eyes. "I see success and long life."

"Well, that's what everyone likes to hear." He takes his ring and stands ready to leave already feeling foolish but relieved by her conclusion he's not dealing with ghosts.

"But I have more."

Daniel eyes a beautiful crystal among her shelf of for sale items. "How much is that crystal?"

"For you Mr. Daniel, $45."

"I'll take it." She wraps it and places it in his hands. Daniel, anxious to leave, approaches the door.

"You'll find what you're seeking," Lydia speaks knowingly.

Daniel stops and turns "Thank you. That was my mother's last wish." He departs knowing he's just tampered with the forbidden teachings he learned in Sunday school but with one less worry- he's not seeing ghosts. It would've shook his belief system for Daniel never believed in them.

Now one more stop. He walks toward the Church of Prophecy a bit cynical of the price he'll be asked to donate there. The building could use some paint and handy work. A landscaper was trimming the brush around the entry way to the short steps of the quaint chapel.

"Is the pastor available?" asks Daniel.

"Yessuh, just mosey on in. He loves greetin' new folk."

"Thanks." Daniel steps inside to see a few rows of pews, some faded curtains, a simple altar, and a few lit candles. He felt good about entering a church -first time in years. Michelle would try and get him to go, but when he did, disappointment was all he could feel, though he did enjoy the dressing up with her to go. Suddenly, he pictured her waiting for him, as she did at their wedding. *What a beautiful bride.* Suddenly he checks his ring finger then sighs a relief that it was there on his finger instead of the fortune tellers. Come to think of it, the ring did feel warm and special. From behind the pew, a piano begins to play and a young girl stands by practicing a hymn.

A middle-aged black man sets out some books by the pulpit and notices Daniel. He then approaches with a big smile and out-reached hand. "God bless you. I'm Pastor Riley."

"Daniel," as they shake hands. Daniel was quick to the point, "Can you foretell the future?"

The pastor chuckles "Have you met Miss Lydia next door? Folks find it funny, I suppose I can't blame them."

"It is rather uncanny, but let's face it, competition is out there." Daniel teases.

'Well, it's a denominational thing, we're in several states. God does know our future and what's the best path.

I have been given certain prophetic visions but mostly we stick with our present lives. Enough problems and rejoicing to go around just in one day," he smiles big.

"And in our past. My mother recently died. I was wondering if you ever witnessed any highly unusual or abnormal behavior during the grieving process, say, among your experiences with parishioners?"

The pastor sensed a need for some personal inspiration and is always ready to hear God for an answer. He gestures to Daniel and they both sit in a pew. "I'm so sorry for your loss. Especially one as close as your mother." The pastor is searching his mental perception but decides to ask directly rather than guess, "What seems to be the disturbing behavior, aside from the pain, of course?"

"My back yard is full of Civil War soldiers. One died in my arms, whose grave was marked over 150 years ago, which I discovered near my mother's grave. The dead are dead are they not?"

Pastor Riley is a bit taken aback. "Yes, most certainly. We have no contact with the dead."

"Then who am I talking to? What am I dealing with? They are certainly real to me."

"Do you have a support group or a church you attend?"

"Just a psychiatrist, and my wife, whom I dare not speak of these things, at least not yet. Please tell me it will go away? I want my life back. Is this some lesson from God?"

"Perhaps, spending some time in prayer and fasting," the pastor suggested, just as perplexed as Daniel is.

"But, you've never run across this type of experience?"

"No, sir. People dwell on the past for a while, but... usually their past with loved ones they miss." Pastor Riley pauses with concern for a moment. "You're not suicidal are you Daniel?"

"No, but how crazy does one have to get before you go there? I have everything to live for, but I must admit I ache terribly in my heart area." Daniel lowers his head into his hands and begins to cry. The pastor puts his arm around him.

"Could you pray for me?" Daniel asks through a few stifled sobs.

"Of, course. God hears our prayers." The pastor softly prays until Daniel's tears come to an end. He feels a sweet calm. Outside it begins to drizzle. There is peace again, if only temporary.

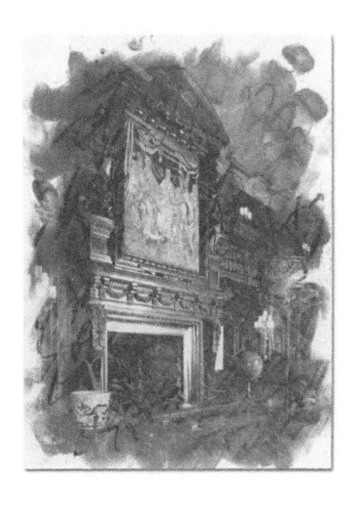

Tick Tock

Nearing the plantation manor just before sunset, the time portal has now crept past the creek and into Daniel's home.

Daniel pulls up and parks at the end of his long driveway, as he eerily senses a foreign presence. He slowly enters the house. He's astounded at what he sees, and a bit overcome with sensory overload. To say his furniture and items have morphed into antiques, as if it were 150 years ago, would be an understatement. Pictured before him would be the envy of the best major film set designer – an award-winning masterpiece! Beginning his visual tour stands out a giant, mantled fireplace, with wood neatly stacked, aglow with slightly crackling knee-high flame, encircled by an area of seating vanities, an overstuffed reading chair, and a richly red, ornately carved, Victorian sofa as if waiting for the Queen. Above the mantle, a large romantic period oil depicting a festivity of poetic looking figures Daniel recognizes as from the Pre- Raphaelite period, not so much lit by the fire but by the wall-to-wall lanterns. Wool blankets, handmade quilts folded nearby, and more laced fine accessories, in an exhibition of comfort readying for winter.

He musters the energy to come out of the coma of wonderment and takes a step. He walks to the dining area, already set for royal guests with seating for twelve. It is laid out with beautiful hand-painted China, framed by decorative silverware and detailed crystal ware. A dazzling chandelier catches his eye above the grand foyer entry way, centered among more Victorian period paintings, with handcrafted elaborate frames, scenes of hunting, stylish picnics, and admiring women strolling under silk umbrellas. He peeks in the kitchen – there are chopping blocks, pans hanging and cookware galore, as if everything was hand-prepared; a wood-burning stove, icebox, and a pantry with no end to it, fully stocked from shelf to shelf. He goes up the half-spiral staircase into his bedroom and finds a beautiful poster bed with a canopy, matching period dresser and night stand, all with marble tops. He opens his closet behind a dressing screen to find men's clothing fit for a Vanderbilt.

Abruptly, he hears a phone RINGING. *I'll snap out of this now! Yes, surely, it's a dream!* Oh, wait; he recalls a small area downstairs still yet unaffected. The land line! Daniel dashes down to the great room, fumbles underneath what's left of modern decor and finds the RINGING phone. It's falling apart but still working.

"Hello," greets a highly anticipatory Daniel.

Sheila Fitzgerald is holding her cell phone in the countryside by a property sign listing: FOR SALE – HOME ON HISTORICAL PLANTATION ACREAGE.

"Sheila Fitzgerald, I hope I'm not imposing. What I have is a wonderful piece of property. It has just been put on the market. It's on a beautiful, former plantation historical site with a contemporary home. Lots of acreage with rows of fruit trees, rolling hills of wildflowers, a classic old barn, a running creek - why you can still even see the remaining original smoke stacks. Oh Mr. Daniel, it is so rich with history. When it went on the market, I immediately thought of you. It would make a dandy investment."

"Dandy? Right now, a dandy place for me would be a high-rise in downtown Manhattan with a Martini bar." Daniel looks around; he notices an annoying TICKING grandfather clock. TICK TOCK. He glances through a window in disbelief as he squints to see outside, the phone still by one ear. TICK TOCK. Irritated by all the goings on, he grabs a crystal carafe half full of liquor in one hand and a glass in the other hand, pressing the cordless phone under his chin, and bolts upstairs.

Miss Fitzgerald understandingly regroups. "I'm so sorry Mr. Daniel; you must still be grieving, perhaps another time?"

"You can say that again!" he exclaims, grateful for an exit opportunity.

Concerned, and slightly confused, she now can't quite hear clearly, "I'm hearing a lot of static. We're having a bad connection. Hello?"

He walks out on the former deck through what is now a set of French doors onto a grand, sweeping balcony. There are sojourners below and covered wagons with an overload of belongings going down his trail along the creek. It appears to be a major route, possibly part of the Underground Railroad, but certainly well-traveled regardless of what it is. His grand balcony is a half-circle of thick, white railing over-and-under Greek revival columns, which is now the new frontage of an ostentatious plantation. He pours a drink and slams it.

Gulping, "Miss Fitzgerald, is there something you're not telling me?"

"Well, I should tell you, that it's probably about $100,000 priced over value. However, the owner has run into hard times."

Staring out the window Daniel snaps, "Give me some time to think about it, say... a couple of hundred years."

The phone call is interrupted amidst the static. It turns into a hodgepodge of wires dangling in his hand which is now completely disconnected. He panics wondering if now there's even an outside world left.

Miss Fitzgerald sympathizes with Daniel, *That poor man. I can just imagine what he's going through.*

Daniel plops onto a sofa in the Great Room. While staring into the fire, time begins to burn itself upon him. *How will I spend my nights? Shall the nights become even longer? My sweet Michelle, this isn't right. I should just walk out of this world, if I even can.*

I am a mere writer. I'm used to relying on my imagination to stimulate and create my world. Now an imaginary world has found me. How uncanny, I've created so many characters, I'm now the lead. However, one noticeable difference – I'm completely powerless!

Daniel drifts into the fire unable to move. *Cheer up. After all, it's only writer's block driving me mad. I still have my pen and paper to stare at while I drink.* He takes a drink straight from the carafe now. *I'll play along with this silly game … until I find out just what the hell is going on.* TICK TOCK.

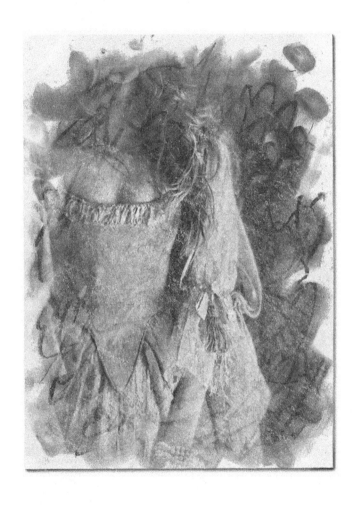

Finding Sarah

The once back acreage dawns to a well-gardened frontage of a grand, Classic Greek Revival plantation, the envy of every passerby.

Daniel walks out dressed like an 1800's upper class gentleman. He steps down in a tightly tailored vest with a pocket watch chain exposed, now attached to the broken watch he found, a silk puff tie, and a white Edwardian shirt underneath an Emerson Frock coat and pants. He stops to gather a few early autumns by the stems and inserts them inside his journal.

A rather well-built bridge fit for walking and horses has replaced a dead log across the creek, which Daniel had earlier wedged to make a temporary crossing. He strolls over and stops midway to immerse his senses below in the clear, refreshing subtle world only nature can provide. His sensations are filled after a slow deep breath, but his thoughts interfere and spoil the moment. Recalling what Brandy had pointed out the day before as "the main cause of such massive death at Andersonville."

A creek; a damned creek – a source for life and cleansing - turned to slow death and filth. Such a betrayal of creation – how could this be? How they must've opened their mouths begging. Oh, but for a drop of rain crying out for mercy with such thirst as the tormented beggar from hell! I don't know if I can ever look at a creek the same. As one views a river that floods to take away a loved one, only the next day, to see it return to peace and calm, leaving no evidence of what it has ravaged in the current.

He tosses a golden leaf from his journal into the flowing stream and wishes his mother could be here, then heads for the stones of Franklin Moore.

Shortly, he arrives at the rock pile memorial then he kneels in silence just staring. The forest of trees seems to join in. He begins writing in his journal:

I have come this day to pay you tribute, young brave soldier. So alone, with no epitaph to reveal that a real genuine soul who loved and was loved lies beneath these stones. I swear by the death of my own mother... (sighs as he writes) *...I will see to it that you get your name back in the land of the living to be restored to honor and dignity.*

He stands and sees a yellow wild flower and places it by the stones and walks away. He starts afoot more inland when he notices a small shed in the thinning woods. He steps on leaf-covered ground another 200 feet. Curious, he goes ever slowly, then opens a door. Straight away, he's startled with a Bowie knife in his face! Daniel falls to the ground on his back, shaken. A black slave is poised in a bravely alarmed stance, gripping the deadly weapon, protecting a young white girl standing in the dimly lit corner. She's gripping something in her arms while herself shivering cold.

Daniel in stroking breaths, but calmly, assures the man to, "Take it easy. I'm not going to hurt you."

Daniel stands, then backs out of the darkened doorway and brushes himself off, watching the slave holding the knife, his chest still breathing hard, without saying anything. He looks Daniel over then back at her. She steps forward into the light, revealing long, wavy blonde hair flowing over her shoulder, clutching a baby close to her. Her eyes look up, catching the light, their color bluer than the sky. Such white skin, soft and fragile - she can't be more than twenty, thin but healthy looking, presuming she's been stranded in these elements.

"What's going on here? Who are you afraid of?" Daniel inquires.

The young girl steps forward, looking Daniel over with less fear, but with one main observation. "You're a Northerner," in her sweet, soft Southern voice, she speaks the truth.

The baby starts whimpering.

"They're all gone now. No Rebs. No Yankees," Daniel insures.

Seeing her white embroidered wear is shear, worn, and insufficient, he takes his long coat off and offers it to her. She looks at the slave, who nods his head, but holds firm. She steps toward Daniel, allowing him to quickly wrap the coat around her. They exchange a close glance, then she steps back.

"Oh, that's a welcome comfort. I have not seen such kindness since my husband marched off to this dreaded war. Ceptin' my slave here, Marcus."

"Yes, Miss Sarah," Marcus humbles himself to show her position.

Daniel is taken to her. "You both should get out of this damp. This shed's no place to be with a baby." He smiles. "Miss Sarah, Marcus. I have accommodations."

She looks at him with hope. Marcus lowers the knife, and then looks at her.

"Fetch my things, Marcus. We shant be staying here this night."

"Yes, Miss Sarah," a relieved Marcus agrees. He puts the Bowie knife inside his pants and picks up a small satchel bag. She smiles with charm at Daniel.

"And who do we owe this debt of gratitude?"

"Daniel. I'm just across the creek," looking back, "I hope."

"My daddy never spoke of no Daniel. You got a family name? Then again, we've drifted so long haven't we Marcus."

Marcus is muscular, about mid-thirties, wearing a white tattered shirt and dark pants with a rope for a belt and no shoes. He puts on a worn hat. Then he finally speaks a full sentence, surprising Daniel of his partially-educated grammar, mixed with country style.

"Yes ma'am. We've been away for a spell. Mr. Daniel is sure a sight. I ain't seen no Northern folk ever before."

They walk to the creek and Marcus follows while holding the baby as Daniel escorts her across the bridge. She eyes the house as they approach. Daniel now realizes the front of the house, once his back acreage, is now facing him in all its grand plantation splendor. He pauses for a moment in wonder. It has fully blossomed into an aristocratic, wealthy estate.

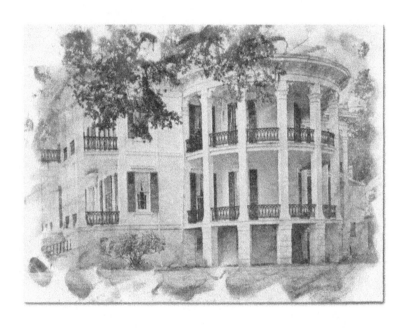

I Own a Plantation

Sarah's eyes widen as if they could get any more noticeable.

"Why, Mr. Daniel, if you have a warm bath inside, then I do believe I'm staring at heaven."

Daniel enchanted, "And I an angel."

She smiles. They go upstairs to the grand veranda porch area, but Marcus stays put at the bottom. Daniel is about to step through the front door when he notices.

"What's he doing?" he asks Sarah.

Sarah with a surprised look at Daniel, "He's not permitted inside another slave owner's house. Surely you have a house slave?"

Daniel is disquieted, then quick to reply, "I could sure use one. Can he cook?"

Sarah calls while grinning, "Marcus. The gentleman asks if you can cook?"

His demeanor becomes animated and he shoots upstairs.

Marcus pitching, "Oh yessuh. I can hunt, skin, cook, fry, bake and make you so fat and spoil you so you can never get up outta that chair to eat my famous Louisiana Mocha Mud Pie. And if my Candied Lemon with Lavender Clafoutis don't make your lips smackin' loud, well suh, my name isn't Marquis De La Jacque Dupre."

A bit wowed, Daniel can't resist. "If we survive this war, I'll have my agent book you a spot on the cooking channel. Come on inside."

Inside the grand foyer, Daniel directs Marcus to the kitchen.

"Marcus, I believe the kitchen is that way...or not. Make yourself at home."

A confused Marcus with that last remark stopped to clarify, "Sir?"

Daniel is struck. "It's an expression. It means, while you stay here, my home is your home."

Marcus takes his hat off and tears up. "You sho a mighty fine man, Mr. Daniel, yessuh. My eyes are so weary of the ugly things in this world, I was beginin' to die inside."

Daniel feels good in this situation. Renewed by her youth and his humble gratitude, he takes the baby from Sarah as they turn and climb the grand staircase.

"And I'm beginning to feel like a lady again." She laughs and kicks off her shoes, drops her bag, and runs barefoot to the top and on up through the house.

Daniel is delighted and feeling ageless. He reaches down for the dropped bag and notices a revolver sticking out. He holds it up and says to the baby, "You have the most enchanting mother."

Daniel walks down the hallway gallery of exquisite Victorian paintings and European baroque tapestries and furniture. *My God, I could live in this hallway.*

He hears Sarah romping and giggling. He walks a bit closer toward her amusing sounds, while carrying the baby and her cloth satchel. He turns into a large master guest bedroom. Velvet red curtains and Elizabethan decor sets the theme of this lavish bedroom. She's jumping on the canopy bed and flopping on her back. She sits up straight when she sees Daniel and gives this look of being found guilty, but full of childlike expression.

"Oh Mr. Daniel Sir, please say these are my sleeping quarters!"

"I'm in the middle of redecorating, but if you insist."

She reaches out for him to bring the baby. When he approaches and holds the child out, she grabs Daniel and hugs him. Then looks sweetly at her baby and says, "Baby Claire, we have a home."

He sits on the bed. "Claire. My, such a lovely name."

"She is named after my dear grandmother. She would've loved this child so, like she so loved me. Do you have a wife, Mr. Daniel?"

He ponders and looks around at his new palatial surroundings. "Not at this particular time."

He stands and straightens his attire. "Sarah, you must be hungry. How have you managed?"

"Oh dear, I almost forgot I was starving. Sir, it's all so difficult this survival thing, must we talk about that now?"

"'Course not. Let's start that bath in heaven."

"Yes! By all means," she beams.

Daniel leaves and walks past room after room of beautiful décor and finally views what appears to be a parlor. He walks in and observes a large, ornate mirror above a vanity, full of sorted bottles, perfumes, and powders that oddly occurs to him how everything is perfectly appointed. Two high-back velvet Victorian chairs with gold trim on one side of the room, a fainting couch and a large tub, beckoning for a bath to be drawn on the other side, pleases the eye. There's a hand pump near a sink with a large bowl and a pitcher on top of a stove, still slightly glowing with heat. He walks around, questioning everywhere his eye pans. He now looks and turns as if he can't find something.

"Oh my God! There's no... oh, hell no!"

He reaches for one last door hoping to discover it.

Relieved, he's thinking *Ah, a toilet fixture. It just needs a magazine rack and some Charmin to complete its usefulness.*

Outside the plantation frontage, a handsome Union Captain with two other soldiers sits on a horse in front of the manor. The upstairs balcony double doors are open. He then starts shouting, "The United States Army, 15th Corps, under Major General William T. Sherman, 53rd regiment Indiana, Captain Stillwater commanding, requests the attention and presence of this plantation manor."

Daniel is pouring more hot water almost filling the bath when Sarah bursts in hysterical. "I just knew this was all just a fantasy dream. Some cruel spell this world is casting upon us."

Daniel is startled that Sarah is referring to witchcraft, which has crossed his mind concerning the time portal, but he's more concerned about the immediate situation, and her nervous outburst.

"Whoa, slow down. What are you talking about?" he asks her.

She grabs him by the hand and leads him down the hallway to the balcony and points outside, carefully tucking into the corridor wall, so as not to be seen.

Stillwater commands, "You sir…"

Daniel steps out while the Captain catches a glimpse of Sarah.

"Are you the owner of this here plantation?"

Daniel proudly declares, "I am."

"In a few days you will be in occupied United States territory. All we ask is that you cooperate with the Union of the States Army as we pass through and volunteer any food and blankets you can spare."

"That sounds fair." Daniel sees an opportunity. "Could you be so kind as to wire a telegraph for me?"

"By all means, as long as you're not telegraphing the enemy," Stillwater responds, only half joking.

"I assure you my intentions are quite the opposite. I'll send down my servant."

Daniel calls Marcus. He writes a quick note.

"Yes, suh…"

Daniel hands him the note addressed to Mrs. Moore.

"Could you please give this to the Captain?"

Marcus looks down at the Union Soldiers somewhat unsure of what to think of this situation. Things were rapidly changing his life. Never the less, he trusts Mr. Daniel so takes the note and delivers it.

Stillwater eyes a peeking Sarah, then looks back at Daniel, who's returned above to the edge of the balcony. Concerning Daniel's manner, he expresses his instinct of his origin and also to make an impression upon such a lovely young woman that she has nothing to fear.

"Why, I perceive you're not a Southerner, Mr.…?

"Daniel. That's right. My ancestor is a Union Sergeant." Sarah steps out into view. "My guest, Miss Sarah."

The Captain takes off his hat and acknowledges her presence with a gentlemanly gesture.

"That be the case Mr. Daniel, I can assign you, Miss Sarah, and your family dutiful guard in the future as things may get, shall we say in the presence of a lady, a bit disagreeable."

He then looks back over the creek at the wooded area and field running uphill.

"You have good ground, especially, that hill beyond - Sugar Hill, according to my map. I'm also scouting for camp sites. I see someone has made use of your land already. I trust you didn't aid them. We'll let you know when we return."

Sarah walks up next to Daniel and holds his arm as the handsome Captain eyes her. He puts his hat on and tips it. "Good day, sir, Ma'am".

They trot down the trail then Daniel puts his arm around her.

"You have nothing to fear. But you're right, this is all just a fantasy - a dream."

Above the estate and the world from another time, the same sun changes light to reflect the day passing from above the modern side, only a few feet, but a phenomenal century and a half later. How can this be, and for what purpose is this window given to Daniel? This thought lulls him to nap on what is now his favorite lounge sofa on the balcony.

"Dinnuh is served," Marcus shouts.

Along the plantation manor frontage on a late afternoon, a few travelers on foot pass by along the trail. Inside the dining room the three occupants are getting acquainted. They're seated over a finished meal of pork, vegetables, and potatoes. Sarah dabs her mouth with a cloth napkin and Daniel pulls out a cigar from his travel with Brandy. Marcus is tending to the baby.

Sarah leans back, "Marcus, if I didn't know your cookin' was so fine and I weren't as hungry as a horse, why I'd never left that bath. Thank you for that moment of enjoyment and this delightful dinner, Mr. Daniel."

Sarah pulls out a watch from her dress knitted pocket and observes the time.

Daniel pulls his napkin from his lap and places it on the table. He is then instantly struck by her pocket watch. He reaches his vest pocket for his and realizes it's missing.

"May I see your watch?"

She hands it to him proudly. Daniel is confounded. To his dismay, it appears to be the identical watch he originally found by the creek with the broken crystal.

"It was my father's watch. The only memento I have from him," she reveals.

She notices a perplexed look on his face as he hands it back to her.

"Would you care to join me out on the veranda, Miss Sarah? Marcus, I'd be willing to guess there is a bottle of Brandy somewhere."

Marcus amuses, "Why Mr. Daniel, you know you have a full liquor cabinet and a wine cellar."

"I have a wine cellar?" Daniel asks impressed.

Marcus sets the sleeping Claire in a makeshift basket then leaves the room. Daniel moves behind Sarah to pull out her chair. They walk out to the veranda then approach the rail and look out upon the grandeur of the grounds.

Sarah sighs a deep breath. "My, the weather has turned to warm the body, and my heart."

"Sarah, I've noticed your way with words, you're an educated girl."

Marcus walks out with a bottle of Brandy on a tray with glasses and a pitcher of water. He sets it on the table and leaves. Daniel pours and offers Sarah. She holds her hand to indicate, 'no thank you.'

Sarah reflecting, "Those were better days. I was cared for and tutored by daddy's travels abroad from the time I was 10 years old, and that seems a lifetime ago, for I am just turned 22. He sent me to my aunt in Virginia at 17, to attend school."

Daniel lights his cigar and takes a swig of the warm liquor.

She continues, "That's where I met my dear husband - at a military ball. He was on leave from West Point, visiting family. He swooned me all the way back to New York where we were married."

"The baby's father?" Daniel inquired.

Sarah bows her head and says nothing. "I believe I will have that drink."

Daniel senses a story as he then pours. "Well, your father must have been proud of you," Daniel assumes.

She holds her glass with both hands and drinks. "Too proud," she begins gasping, almost choking from the warm, potent alcohol. She catches her breath after that drink. Daniel exhales his cigar then pours her some water.

"Thank you. Pride is a two-edged sword, Mr. Daniel. His pride educated me, but nearly destroyed me."

With sarcasm, she exclaims, 'My husband is a damned Yankee!" Gathering her strength "Yes, from Virginia, but when this detestable war started, he had to choose. For General Lee, it was honorable, for my Jonathan, he was a traitor in my daddy's eyes. Now I don't know what's become of my soul, or my husband."

She starts tearing up. Daniel wants to hold her, but resists, and observes her pain. His wisdom tells him in thought not to immediately rescue a woman from her tears. *Men want to instinctively put their arm around them and relieve her. That merely prevents her need to cry fully. She needs to feel and process her pain, let her cry. She will come to you to be held when ready. Hmm...yet there's a time when validation and comfort consoles the soul. Which does she need from me?*

Sarah, now crying, offers, "Please forgive me, but I must retire. I'm in need of some long overdue sleep."

Daniel sets down his drink. "That's completely understandable."

He starts to sit when suddenly she returns wiping her tears.

"I feel safe with you. Thank you kindly".

She hugs him tightly as he responds with his arms, then slips away. Daniel wonders what his role is with her. He sits down and has another drink, puts his feet up on the railing and continues to enjoy his cigar. Owls start hooting, squirrels play high in the limbs. The wind picks up and a few more turning leaves begin to spin as they fall to the ground. Daniel surmises, *This has been the most splendid day. I'm beginning to enjoy this time menagerie. What's there to fear? Never coming back?*

Later, in his voluminous master bedroom, he writes that down in is his journal before he forgets that feeling. While lying in silk pajamas and a long robe, he ponders the whole experience as of late.

Daniel Journals:

> *Perhaps time itself is the illusion and is not really passing by at all.*

He picks up a glass sitting by a Kentucky Whiskey bottle and takes a drink.

> *I have found that I am rather gifted at this calligraphy style, my pen just flows.*

He pauses.

> *Sarah. Whatever am I to make of her? Her body language tells me there's a story behind her lady-like facade. When I asked her about her child - she's but a child herself. Oh, Sarah, I do fancy the child in you.*

He laughs. *My God, I sound like a romantic Southern gentleman.*

Marcus clears his throat, "Is there anything I can get you before I retire sir?"

Daniel turns to see Marcus at the open doorway.

"You know you're a free man here, Marcus."

"No suh. As long as Miss Sarah needs me, that's as free as I be."

"Is she sleeping?"

Marcus chuckles, "Why that girl can sleep through a cannon ball a blazin...septin when she has them nightmahs, Lord knows."

"About her husband?"

Marcus looks down, then up. "I reckon she'll talk about it, when time comes."

Daniel looks concerned. "Is there anything I can do?"

"She'll be fine in the morn. She loves my pancake fixins. That's what I need to ask, suh, well, you'll be needin more kitchen goods. You know, til I can get some huntin' done. When that officer said, 'volunteer food'...he means he's coming back for lots a food."

Daniel snaps, "Food. Supplies. Military Guests. Sure, what was I thinking? You must think I run a low budget mansion here. I'll get on it."

Marcus looks at him sort of surreal. "Yesuh. Good night, suh."

"Good night." As Marcus leaves the room, he leans his forehead on his hand, *Darn, I gotta make a midnight run to Walmart.*

The all- night Walmart is practically empty. Daniel loads up on food and baby supplies. He scratches his head over things like coffee, so he loads up with cans of it. He then piles one whole cart with bacon, hamburger and hot dogs. He figures Marcus can make bread from what he saw in the pantry and find farm vegetables including potatoes and corn from nearby. He walks through the aisle of magazines, one with Civil War articles, and can't help but grab a few. As he's standing in line with three carts, he glances over at a giant Teddy bear sitting at a toy kiosk and contemplates bringing it home.

It's now 2 A.M. after a quick 'manly' in and out shopping spree, Daniel drives by the open Waffle House and decides to grab a bite.

Why not?

When he circles around to park, he sees Donna trying to start her car. He pulls next to her and gets out.

"Sounds like you have a problem."

She recognizes him and half-smiles to see him.

"Hi. It's my fault. I let the gas get too low," Donna says in a frustrating way. She gets out of her car, looks at her watch.

"Real smart," she sighs. "My kids will be worried...my cell is dead..."

"How far do you live from here?"

"About 15 minutes."

"It's too late and you're too tired. Hop in."

Inside his car, he notices she has cigarettes. He can tell that she's a single mother. In one of his novels he did a lot of research on single parenting. He understood it's a lonely and hard life, especially for someone who's struggling financially. Perhaps one of his own fears for having children, that someday they may not have two parents. He looked at her hands that didn't quite match the rest of her soft, ebony skin throughout her face and arms. She's managed to keep her nails and probably could've been a model years ago. There may have been a time where she did look much younger than her age but now that it's catching up to her. He wants her to feel comfortable.

"You can light up if you like."

"Oh, thank you. I need to unwind. I don't like this shift. I was filling in for someone. Last minute favor." She looks over at him after she lights up, feeling curious. "You been out night clubbin?"

He smiles. "Not exactly."

She looks in the back and sees the food. "My, you've got enough bacon to feed an army."

"You could say that again."

They laugh together.

The car winds down a dimly lit road, typical for rural Georgia. Donna wants to ask him a lot of questions, especially about what he does, but even more, as to what motivates him. After all, he did awaken in her that dormant desire, *I want more out of life. Do I have what it takes to change?* She remembers pondering after their first meet, to dig deeper as to what really drives her. She is building the courage to talk to him about it. *I don't want to pester him with questions, that's what nagging wives do*, she thought.

They pull up to her house and remain inside his car.

Donna lifts her feet up to her seat and starts rubbing "My feet are going to love that bed."

He turns off the engine as she looks over at him feeling a bit cozier.

"You asked me if I was happy, remember?"

"Now I do."

"I've done a lot of thinking since you asked me that. I'm thinking of taking some classes, you know, to better myself. I've been so dedicated to my daughters and making ends meet, I've hardly had time for myself."

Daniel likes the appreciation that she listened to him. It was his first attraction to Michelle.

"That takes some drive and courage," Daniel responds.

His validation and complement has taken her to a new level of comfort with him.

"Did you ask because you care about me?" she searches.

"I was having a moment," he says honestly. "You became part of it."

"Can you be happy and still be lonely?" Silence. She leans over and kisses him lightly on the lips.

"Now, you have me thinking," he says, feeling more awkward about the kiss than the question.

Her teen child steps out into the porch light as the screen door shuts.

"It's late," Donna says softly. "Thank you so much. Maybe we can pick this up where we left off another time."

"Another time perhaps." *If she only knew...*

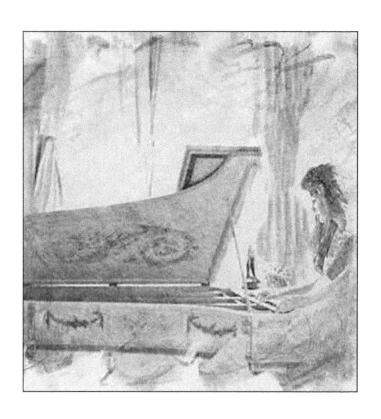

Mourning Sonata

It's early morning. Lovely piano music is coming from somewhere. Moonlight Sonata by Beethoven.

Daniel rises and puts on his robe. He floats down the gallery hallway, drawn to the beautiful notes, an evocative echo. Daniel descends the grand stairway into the foyer. Music fills the air throughout, like a magic ethereal presence. He notices the open door to the Great Room.

The burgundy felt walls with high ceiling, detailed with hand-carved molding, make for a splendid acoustic surrounding. An oil mural, depicting an English countryside, fills an entire wall. Baroque period tapestries are everywhere, surrounding European fine cabinets with colored glass and a large roll top desk, which is anchored below an early impressionist painting.

He enters the room and finds Sarah playing on a large white grand piano. The sunlight streaming through the curved glass, framed in velvet curtains, is glowing off her hair and gown. Daniel's senses are filled as he sits and listens, mesmerized by it all. On the table before him is an envelope with an open letter beside it. He picks it up and reads.

April 6, 1864

Mrs. Jonathan A. Saunders,

Respected lady, I feel it is my duty to send you a few lines. It is with great sorrow that I tell you that your husband Jonathan A. Saunders of my company, sent out on detail from Canton, Mississippi, on the 28th day of March 1864, has not returned. There has been no word since. He has always been a good soldier and very ready as a leader, and I was sorry to lose him from the company. Yours truly, Captain Samuel Evans.

Daniel sees a stack of letters from her husband tied in a red ribbon. She stops playing.

"Sarah, how long have you known?"

Sarah looks out into the light. "About a month after the date on that letter. My aunt in Atlanta had Union ties and connections. She inquired."

"Why not delivered to you?"

She turns to Daniel and with all seriousness, and conveys the heart of the matter.

"When I returned home, I was no longer welcome. My father shunned me. I saw a side of him I can't explain. Where was I to go? Mother was ailing. She tried comforting me. "This war won't last," she said, "Your father will come around." After much fretting, we thought it best I stay with her sister in Atlanta. Well, weeks grew into months, then a year. Marcus would bring letters on occasion from Jonathan, at least those my father didn't hide or burn. Then they just stopped. I had no idea where he was."

Daniel puts a log on the fire. He sits listening. She gets up and lingers by the letters, sifting through them reminiscing.

"Sometimes I'd sneak back to see my sickly momma. Bless her soul. When she died, Daddy was heartbroken and took me back in. It was fall last, I believe. That's when I found the letters. Yes, it was about this season, for the leaves had started barely to turn. Jonathan was in Mississippi. It was crazy at the time but my desire was toward nothing but being with him, so I took a train to Vicksburg. Lord, I never seen so many Yankees before. I thought the war must be over."

"You found him?"

"Oh yes. Word traveled fast among those men when I inquired. I'd found a room overlooking the Mississippi and he was given a short leave. I've never known such splendor. My memory is hazy after that, as that is when..." She moves on and walks over to the window. "That was the last time I saw him. He sent one letter to my aunt's address as I suggested that would be better."

Daniel's intuitive senses kick in "There's something you're not telling me, Sarah, which is fine. I'm so sorry about your husband, and your mom." He gets up and walks over to her. "You're safe here for now. I brought you something."

She turns like a child and smiles. "Oh Daniel, show me! At this very moment."

He takes her hand and they walk into the parlor on the main. There, seated in the chair, is a large Teddy bear. She runs over and holds it up, then she hugs it, as Daniel looks on the reaction he was hoping for.

"Wherever did you get such a thing?"

"I'm glad you like him. I think he's hungry, let's get you both something to eat."

"You are the strangest man."

Just then Marcus enters.

"There's a Mrs. Moore here to see you, suh."

Daniel shows a sudden concern with interest.

"I'll need to get dressed. Have her seated in one of these fancy rooms where you can serve us food and tea."

"Yes, suh."

"Excuse me, my lady," he says, leaving Sarah with a curious but respectful look on her face.

Moments later Daniel enters a guest area where a stately woman is seated having tea with a traveling female. When Daniel enters, they both stand as he greets them. "Mrs. Moore, I'm Daniel."

"Emily Moore," she turns "My sister Abigail. I received your telegram. Thank you so kindly. You're positive it was my son?"

Daniel pulls out the letter, Molly's picture, and a few of his belongings in a case. She then turns to her sister and buries her head in her breast and cries. Marcus appears with a tray of food, but Daniel waves him off. *Someone did truly love him.* Daniel's thoughts of Franklin's abandonment at his gravesite are slightly relieved now, but her grief is almost unbearable, watching her hands clutching tighter to the shoulders of her comforting sister. Abigail gently strokes her sister's hair then with tears of her own, looks over at Daniel.

"I've lost a husband and my only brother. I thought I had no tears left, but there seems to be no end. Such a sweet nephew he was."

Mrs. Moore backs away as Abigail hands her a fresh handkerchief. She dabs her eyes then turns to Daniel. "We've disrupted your day Mr. Daniel, please forgive me."

"It's quite understandable. If it's any consolation, he died in my arms while I read your loving letter. He truly missed you." Daniel remembers Molly but refrains from asking. "Would you care for some more tea, perhaps stay for a meal?"

She considers his request. "That is most kind but we must make proper arrangements. I've thought about it on the way here...but I decided if it was truly my Franklin, that I could not bear to walk by his grave every day. If there's a proper cemetery nearby then that will be his final resting place."

"There is," Daniel says, as he envisions that funeral that began this destined journey and has brought their lives together, almost 150 years apart. Time means nothing to him now.

"Good. I hope you do understand my reason Mr. Daniel. If you'll kindly direct me to him, we'll be on our way."

After leaving them at the shallow marker, Daniel later watches from above, out his manor window.

Beethoven's notes are echoing again, more hauntingly now, as Sarah resumes play.

Daniel Journals:

This was the strangest moment of my life. Escorting the heartbroken mother of a too-young-to-die Civil War soldier, only to bury him in a grave he's already been lying in for 150 years. Reality is such a thin line.

Noon day, the plantation manor frontage is quiet and clear. The trees sway in a sudden breeze as the autumn leaves are beginning to cover the ground. His body is taken away by a local undertaker, followed by the two women in a carriage.

DANIEL Journals:

These trees will ever keep the lore, of the ghost of Franklin Moore.

As Daniel later reflects on the veranda, Marcus comments "You did a might kind thing with huh, Mr. Daniel. Yes, suh, no folks care no mo."

"I couldn't have lived with myself, his life seemed of no consequence." *Now, at least to me, I can put a face and a life on that cold stone I saw...what seems, so long ago.*

Daniel is morphing along with the portal. His manner, even the way he speaks is becoming of an early 19th Century aristocratic gentleman. His writing, a blending of past and present, seems to now flow with more ease and creative energy. A newfound purpose perhaps, finding a new man that was always there waiting to be discovered, through grief and death, he felt new life.

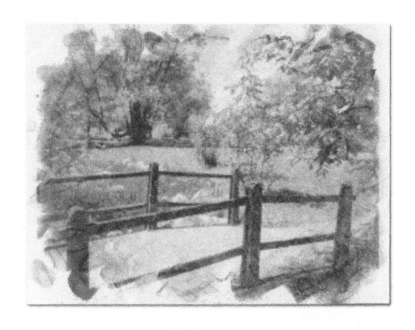

A Slave's Bounty

Later afternoon in the dining room, Marcus fidgets about something. Daniel is seated by his almost empty plate, reading an 18th century leather-bound novel from his library. Sarah has excused herself to feed the baby. Marcus gathers her dishes and reaches for Daniel's as he quickly grabs the last biscuit from the center tray.

Daniel jokingly asks, "Pillsbury or Betty Crocker?"

There is no one to answer, but he amuses himself.

Marcus fumbles with the dishes. "Mr. Daniel, I have to tell you... please suh, I might've done wrong."

Daniel finishes his food and kidding again, "You over cooked the bacon a bit?"

Marcus seems nervous so Daniel senses the tone and sets down his book.

Marcus continues, "I was helpin kin folk...it's just for the night. Please, suh...I'll show you."

Daniel wipes his mouth and puts down the napkin as Marcus leads him outside.

A few hundred feet alongside the manor there's a rustic large shed, the size of half a barn. He rounds the corner, with Daniel trailing.

When Marcus is about to open a door. "What's this?" Daniel asks, perplexed at the structure.

Marcus hesitates, "Why, you know this is your smoke house, suh."

He swings open the door and Daniel sees four pair of big white eyes in the shadows.

"My kin, massuh Daniel, I had no choice. Please, they were going to turn them in to the bounty man."

"I'm not your massuh, Marcus," he blurts out.

Daniel shuts the door and jaunts back to the house while exhibiting an extreme, uncharacteristic side of frustrating anger. Marcus runs behind, then Daniel swiftly turns to face him.

"You mean a slave bounty?" Daniel knows enough history to understand the severity.

"Yes, suh."

Aggravated by this turn of events, he spills more out, "My life just got too complicated." Looking up, he asks, "This is what I get for not having children? A bunch of slaves?" As Daniel walks away, he sternly insists, "Feed them and send them on their way, Marcus."

Marcus stops a bit surprised. "Yesuh. Right away. Please forgive me." He heads back to the shed.

Daniel's hot button surfaces without restraint. His aversion to caring for the helpless needs of others - a responsibility he feels he cannot live up to, at least more than himself, a self-justified reason for putting off his late marriage. Hence, children and pets have also remained out of the picture. Marcus was certainly an asset and self-reliant, and Sarah, a child who'd come of age, but a house full of slaves? It just unexpectedly overwhelmed his weakness. A flaw he just wasn't ready to address. In the portal with slaves or in the life he was escaping with Michelle wanting a child. Perhaps he was getting too comfortable. *Why does this always seem to happen when I find that place of peace with myself?* he wondered.

Daniel doesn't even get inside the door when the sound of horses and three riders approach, pulling a slave by a rope. Daniel turns and freezes. The main rider, dressed in a period black trench coat and a short top hat, approaches, pulling the slave as the other two nasty looking ones stand back.

The lead bounty man turns to the slave "Is that him? Is this the place?"

The slave nods his head yes and bows looking down. This was no ordinary bounty man. Rufus Jones had a reputation the slaves feared the most in all this territory. Stories of setting men and women on fire to get them to talk was well known. Marcus was now trapped with the others inside the shed.

Rufus now narrows in on Daniel "You best tell me now where them Nigger slaves is cuz if we hafta' go lookin' and find them we'll burn this house to the ground."

Daniel steps to the edge, staring as if he's seen the genuine face of evil for the first time.

"Your manners are barbaric," he stares him squarely in the face. "I suggest you get off my property."

Rufus, faster than the eyes can see, pulls out a whip and lashes the slave who falls to the ground. "The next one's for you. Start searchin' boys. We're gonna' show 'em the devil. Bo, you get the barn."

Marcus comes screaming out of the smokehouse, "Stop! I'm the one. Take me. I did it."

Bo gets off the horse and knocks Marcus to the ground. Marcus looks at Daniel with a bloody mouth and painful eyes, drawing Daniel to approach him when Marcus holds up his hand. "No suh. He means it, Mr. Daniel. Please stop. We'll go."

Daniel looks over the situation as the three male slaves and one female are led out by Bo the bounty as Rufus instructed.

"We got 'em," Bo says satisfied.

The sinister Rufus, remaining on his horse, looks at Daniel with a malevolent smile that would creep a fierce dog into hiding. "I'm bounty Rufus C. Jones, and you are messin' with my money. These niggers are my valuables, and you suh, are a thief and conductor on this here operation and will not be tolerated."

He's referring, unbeknownst to Daniel, of the Underground Railroad, the name given to the secret network of passageways and safe houses whereby slaves escaped to freedom...or death.

Bo suggests with zeal, "Let's hang em."

"That won't be necessary. What's your bounty?" Daniel appeals.

Rufus stares and answers after he spits, "250 dollars in U.S. or gold."

"I'll pay you $250, plus a $100 for the man on the rope."

Rufus thinks about it, then takes the rope off the slave's neck. "Deal," as he spits again on the ground near Daniel's feet.

The slave quickly joins the other four but Marcus just stands, suspiciously wondering about this situation. Daniel reaches in his coat inner pocket for his wallet and pays him. As Daniel backs up the stairs, Rufus throws the rope around Marcus' neck. "Those are yours. We're gonna hang this nigger fer hidin' 'em."

He pulls Marcus to the ground while another bounty man throws a rope over a tree branch with a hanging noose. Daniel starts for Marcus but the other slaves stop him and hold him. Bo pulls out a club from his saddle bag. Daniel screams!

Bo eagerly says, "First, we gotta beat him to a pulp." The others laugh.

Daniel shouting viciously, "You murderers! Stop this madness!"

Both men start for Marcus when he suddenly pulls out his Bowie knife and slices the face of one and jabs the other. Rufus quickly whips away his knife causing Marcus to scream with pain. They gag him and wrestle him back to the noose and put it around his neck, then pull until it can't get any tighter, lifting him kicking in the air. Everyone is frozen with horror. All that's heard now is Marcus squirming and strangling heavily. Suddenly, the sound of a gun being cocked is audible above the chaos.

"You turn him lose or I'll send you to hell!"

Rufus turns, flinches his whip then looks down the barrel of an Army Colt revolver as Sarah points it at him from the edge of the veranda. He's in no position to gamble.

Rufus, plotting his next move, gives the orders, "Cut 'em loose."

Marcus is released, dropping to the ground, gasping for air.

Sarah commands, "Get their guns, Marcus."

Marcus staggers a bit then grabs his knife and takes two guns from the men about to hang him. She inches closer to Rufus still from the above vantage, firmly holding the gun with both hands. "Get off your horse."

Marcus has the others on hold while Daniel is let go and stands watching Rufus get down. Her face determined, eye steady on the gun site and body unwavering in her full-length dress. "Say your last words."

Marcus pleads, 'Miss Sarah. These aint the men. Let 'em go."

Daniel wonders what he means.

"He's a raider. Ain't no matter," she answers steadily.

Rufus righteously looks around, "You'll all hang for this."

Unexpectedly, the sound of galloping horses rumble from across the creek as everyone but Sarah turns to see Union Cavalry, led by Captain Stillwater, now clopping over the wooden bridge. He waves his troops to a quick maneuver. They immediately dismount and surround the perimeter, pulling out their rifles and aim. Stillwater pulls up on horseback. "What's all this?"

Sarah boldly says, "They were gonna hang my slave, now I'm gonna shoot him dead."

Stillwater swings one leg over the head of the horse and lands directly in front of Rufus, staring in his eyes. He turns back to Sarah slowly with a grin "That would certainly be doing the Union a favor."

She doesn't flinch. He's admiring her courage then steps closer to her. Poetically, "Beauty always triumphs over beast."

For the first time, she takes her eye off her target to glance at the Captain standing below her, then back aiming sharper at Rufus.

Sarah eerily responds, "Not this kind of beast."

The Captain is a bit chilled by her demeanor. His attempt to release the tension has failed. Sincerely, he attempts to sway Sarah, "He'll get justice. I promise, Miss Sarah. Let him go."

Marcus believes him. "Listen to him Miss Sarah."

She starts a little shaking. Stillwater slowly moves closer to her and gently says, "It's over Sarah."

He reaches out his hand and takes the gun quickly. Daniel takes her as she buries herself in his chest and arms. Rufus starts to mount.

"You stay put," Stillwater firmly demands.

Another small group of Union Cavalry and officers, are now galloping over the bridge with one Major General in their midst, wearing hat, beard, and an obvious charismatic stature. Rufus disregards and continues when Stillwater quickly grabs the reins.

"Let go you Yankee bastard, this war ain't over yet," Rufus threatens.

The General's authoritative voice interjects "Because of fools like you who talk sedition and refuse to face reality…"

They turn and face his commanding presence. The men in direct vicinity move to stand at attention as he continues "…blinded to the fact that you are completely surrounded, outnumbered, out flanked and out gunned by men far superior to you in bravery and in character, if I surmise correctly what is in front of me." He pauses. "At ease."

Rufus is immobilized at this striking personality. Daniel recognizes this man as General Sherman while he watches him put a cigar butt in his mouth.

"You sir, are speaking to one of my finest officers of the Union Army of the United States of America, under my command, General William T. Sherman." He pulls the cigar butt out of his mouth. "Tecumseh. Remember that from your cell. Arrest these men."

"Yes sir." Stillwater motions to the men and they grab the slave bounty hunters. General Sherman walks up the stairs. "Someone be kind enough to show me to my quarters and fetch me some Brandy."

Daniel, not surprised at anything now, waves Marcus to oblige.

Marcus leads the way. "This way, suh."

Stillwater shrugs his shoulders at Daniel, holds out his hand gesturing, 'You first,' and then follows up the stairs.

The estate is bustling with activity and has become the southern hospitality palace it was designed for, accompanying guests from all walks of life. A General and his staff are settling in their new accommodations in an elegant environment while guards stationed throughout, are positioning themselves for any surprise that might disrupt the peace and comfort to which they are unaccustomed. Sarah, now the Southern Belle of the estate, catches their eye as she strolls about the manor dressed to perfection. The smell from the kitchen is drawing attention as Marcus removes his apron and begins preparations for what he hopes to be a special occasion.

Not long after on the second floor, Daniel wearing dressed attire, is standing in front of a dressing mirror, downing a whiskey in his bedroom. *I'm not quite sure the occasion, but I know something is brewing.*

"Massuh Daniel, suh." Marcus politely addresses by the door.

"Come in. You all right?" Daniel responds with genuine concern.

Marcus is also changed into better attire. "Yes, thank you. I owe you my life…and Miss Sarah." He winks at Daniel. "We are ready for you in the servant's quarters."

"I have servant's quarters?"

Beneath the kitchen is a large chamber made of stone that is large enough to store flour sacks, rice, shelves full of tools, beds for 8 and enough area for leisure. There are a few tables and desks lit by lanterns, plus plenty of logs stacked by the fireplace and a cooking stove. There's even a kneeling and prayer area.

The four slaves are all standing in a row wearing proper servants' attire. Marcus and Daniel stand before them as each one steps forward and gives their name.

Mabel yields with a curtsy, "Mabel, suh".

Charles steps forward proudly, with a slight bow, "Charles sir." His obvious proper English education stands out as he steps back, allowing the next to step forward.

Shyly, "Oakley, suh."

He steps back looking down the nudges the next one. "Well, go ahead Boone." Boone looks next in line at William then steps forward last.

"I'z Boone, this here is my brother William, he can't speak."

Marcus leans to Daniel and whispers, "They cut his tongue out."

Boone then adds, "But he can sho speak with his banjo," he remarks.

"We'z so thankful fo whatju did…" says Oakley.

Marcus concludes, "Jackson, the one they dragged here… likes to work with animals and sleep in the barn. Might not see him inside."

Daniel has forgotten his rash irritability at the thought of such selfish resistance turning them away, as he is reminded looking over at the red, blood ring around Marcus' neck. Mabel's watering eyes are holding back her deepest fears – being rejected only to become a fugitive again. And William. the man's tongue had been savagely severed from his throat. Daniel couldn't imagine a speechless life. Charles, he would later learn, was an English freeman, working on a British cargo vessel, when he was taken captive at a Louisiana port and sold into slavery, lured by a black woman. Daniel wonders in thought, *Who could they become, afforded the same interpretation that all men are created equal? A brutal war destined to answer that very purpose. For now, it is bestowed upon me, the power to give them hope or despair. The portal is teaching me I can no longer live within the shallow belief system of my comfortable world, that is, if this is truly the change I am seeking.*

"Massuh, Daniel, suh, you still want to free them and send them on their way, suh?"

"Now that would hardly be freedom, would it Marcus?"

Daniel knows his answer. He walks down the line, feigning he's a stern master. Then stops and turns firmly. "They can stay under three conditions."

Marcus and the servants are at Daniel's full attention. "They accept wages, attend a tutoring session daily at my expense, and read books, mainly the classics."

Marcus looks at Daniel with relief then shakes both Daniel's hands. "You a mighty fine man,"

Daniel smiles. "It's all right if you call me, massuh. It's grown on me rather fondly."

The servants are jubilated.

Afterwards, Daniel steps outside onto the veranda, then down the stairs and walks up to one of the posted guards and hands him a cigar. "I'm taking a walk."

"Thank you. I'll get you escort."

Daniel muses "Don't bother. He might disappear."

Daniel walks around and crosses the time line.

Loud rap music is coming from a distance. He glances up to the house on the hill, then plugs a USB Wi-Fi device into his laptop, from in the back of his SUV. Up pops an email from Michelle. He immediately opens it and sees a selfie of her with a short note. She looks casual and smiling, bringing a warmth over him.

My Dearest Daniel,

I miss you. I've tried calling. Left you messages several times. I'm in between meetings so I'll check my messages after a while. Hopefully, I'll hear your voice telling me you're alright and coming home soon.

Jason keeps calling. What do I tell him? He's invited me over for dinner with Janet. He's even had her

*call me. I'll pick up a bottle of his favorite wine and
tell him it's from you.*

Missing you!
With love,
Michelle

He responds by typing:

Dear Michelle,

*I'm sorry. My phone is having problems. No excuse.
Please be patient. That's a beautiful picture of you.
I am writing again. That's some comfort.* He then
realizes an uncanny resemblance to the exchange
between a wife and husband- loved ones in time
of war, separated by time and space. Some things
never change.

He's interrupted from cars starting their engines, some
pulling away and more arriving. He finishes the email with
a quick "*goodbye, I love you, Daniel*" then pushes send. He
realizes the neighbor is having one of those infamous parties, so he decides to walk up the drive and check out the
alternative lifestyle of the other neighbor.

Upon entering J.J.'s courtyard, the hard-core rap music
becomes louder. The majority are black, some guests are
white, and they are all dancing and mingling. Daniel is
overwhelmed by the contrasting decadence, glaring jewels
and the over-the-top dress apparel, to his humble former
slaves he just left. He sees a few are openly using drugs,
while the booze is flowing. Ambiguous adult acts can be
made out from the dark corners. He looks up at the flag pole

with J.J.'s iconic insignia flying, then walks up to the DJ on the small stage just below.

Daniel makes a request in a loud and self-amusing voice, "Got any Marvin Gaye?"

The deejay keeps grooving then shakes his head and smiles, revealing a big, gold grille. Daniel looks around and eyes a few provocative women being hit on by male clones of rap idols. One is staring down at Daniel rather provokingly. He feels way out of place and moseys back down the driveway. He sees J.J. through the front windshield of an otherwise darkly tinted makeshift bedroom, in the back of a Rolls with two naked girls.

On the upper balcony, Sarah is talking with baby Claire, seemingly much calmer. Stillwater approaches her. "Care if I join you?"

"Please do. I see your men have a great respect for you, Captain. They told me of your bravery on the field of battle. Why, hear them tell it, you and your General have conquered the entire western hemisphere."

He swells like a rooster. "He chooses his battles wisely. We execute with discipline. From what I saw, you're the brave one. I can't help but asking, Miss Sarah... were you going to pull the trigger?"

She sets the sleeping baby in a bassinet. "I assure you, five more seconds and I would've emptied that chamber into his chest. Does that surprise you, Captain Stillwater?"

"I'm not sure it was him you were aiming at." He takes her hand gently and looks at her skin

"These are not the hands of a senseless killer."

Down the hallway gallery, General Sherman is entering the upper parlor for his bath wearing one of Daniel's finer robes. Charles is with him.

Sherman mutters in his usual gruff manor, "I'll be damned if I let war matters keep me any longer from the pleasure of a warm bath and wet Brandy."

Charles feels he's in the presence of a larger than life figure, but can't quite put his finger on what is taking place. He's used to treatment unbecoming a human with any substance. "I'll just pour it again, General, sir, this is steaming hot, as you requested."

"Your manners and service will soon be rewarded, as well as your suffering," Sherman surmises as he sinks into the warm tub.

Hope. That's it, Charles realizes the word he was searching for. That's what he was feeling in Sherman's presence. Hope. He gladly pours as the steam rises. "Yes sir. Perhaps you're right."

Marcus is talking with the others as he prepares for bed in the servant's quarters.

"Lord, these ol' bones is tired. I got to get up early, feedin' that Genril is mighty important."

Boone laughs. "You could be swingin' high from dat' oak tree, cousin. Sho' was a close call today."

"Whatchall laughin' fo', you be swingin' too," Oakley adds.

They all laugh. Marcus looks out, dreaming. "I sho' be glad when my day comes. I'll be cookin' in the finest Lweesana restaurant, folks come for miles to taste my fixins. Yes, suh, chef Marquis de La Jacque DuPre gonna make a name for himself.

Sarah is looking out over the banister of the upper balcony. "You have a wife back home, Captain?"

Stillwater steps closer "No, ma-am. I'm married to the army."

"You're more fortunate. For the army has divorced me from my husband and my family, with nothing to show for it but my childhood past lying in ruins. They were not there when my family needed them."

"I'm sorry to hear. Perhaps I can help you recover some fondness for a man in uniform."

He starts to kiss her.

"A splendid night under the circumstances..." Daniel interrupts from the entry way.

He then steps on to the balcony as they separate.

"...I mean surrounded by war and lawlessness. It is certainly some mysterious providence that has brought us all here together at this place and time. Wouldn't you agree Captain?"

"I assure you as long as we are here, your peace and safety, as well as your abundant prosperity, shall remain."

Sarah relieved, excuses herself, "I shall leave you men to sort out the affairs of divine providence, man and country. After all, what does a woman know of such things? Good night gentlemen."

As she takes the baby and leaves, the way she moves is noted by both men.

"Good night, Sarah," ends Daniel with a tender farewell for the evening.

Stillwater slightly bows, "My lady."

Stillwater continues his point with Daniel, "As I was saying, we will pulverize the enemy. Strike the fear of hell on theses damnable backward Neanderthals and so soak the soil with their blood, then fertilize it with widows and orphans. They'll wish they were never born."

Daniel, a bit aghast, challenges his views, "If that's your version of peace and safety..."

Charles interrupts "Mr. Daniel sir, the General requests your presence in the parlor." Charles remains standing in the doorway.

"Excuse me. Normally I'd say we'll continue this conversation, but I think not," Daniel leaves Stillwater and heads to the parlor.

"Bring me a serving of that pudding pie from supper," Stillwater requests.

"Yes sir." Charles exits.

Stillwater takes a drink, plops his feet on the ledge and revels in his future conquest of the enemy… and of a certain young woman.

General Sherman and The Letter

S herman is laid back in the tub with a short, unlit cigar in his mouth, a glass half full of Brandy on the ledge, while holding a letter down outside the tub.

He welcomes Daniel as he walks in, "Have a seat on one of your plush Victorian chairs." Daniel is seated while he pulls out one of his own cigars, lights it with a stick from the stove coals then likewise lights Sherman's as he begins to puff, "Your manners and character are befitting a Northerner." Sherman complements.

"And yours, befitting a legend."

Sherman chuckles. "Flattery noted. You sir, would make a grand politician - one who leaves the war to those on the battlefield. But then, I flatter with sarcasm, it would be a curse on you and such a one does not exist in Washington, as I just described."

He shakes the letter and continues dryly, "Drat those confounded meddling fools. They fancy a war in peace time and dread war when it's time to annihilate the enemy. Then give orders from Washington before they end the night at one of those high society balls where they are discussing the finer things of...er, more refinement, while slipping out the back to cheat on their wives."

"Well that hasn't changed," Daniel answers sarcastically. He then looks at the letter Sherman is holding, while the General continues his style of philosophical preaching.

"This here letter from the President, not his doing, it's that damnable War Secretary Scranton!"

Daniels eyes widen, "You're holding a letter from President Lincoln?"

Sherman obviously not listening, "Needs another victory before the election? Hell, I just handed him Atlanta and the election victory."

"In the bath tub?" Daniel continues to marvel.

"Damn, if we didn't just walk through Georgia like pissing downwind on Jeff Davis' flag and crushed General Hood in three days. It's now under siege, with more cannon fodder than weighs an ironclad warship!"

"May I see?" Daniel asks.

He hands Daniel the letter, then takes a drink. "Now they want to side track my intentions for the final blow by sending a regiment to Andersonville Prison to get some damn VIP officer who is family to the President."

Daniel looks up from the letter. "Andersonville? My ancestor is a Union Sergeant imprisoned there."

Sherman takes his cigar out and holds the Brandy glass to his mouth. "I hear stories. Dreadful."

Daniel perks up at the opportunity, "They will bury over 13,000 men there, carry out 200 per day, starvation and dysentery is rampant. The food is now almost cut off. The confederates will resort to grinding up corn husks, tearing the soldier's guts out with slivers inside. They wallow in their own feces."

Sherman now alarmed and listening asks, shocked, "How do you know all this?"

"There are 30,000 to 40,000 men there at present in a stockade built to house and feed only 9,000, and only for a short period. The warden, Captain Wirz, will be hanged for war crimes. You sir, will change the course of history and be instrumental the signing of General Lee's surrender with Grant."

Sherman sits up. "Undeniably a desirable foretelling," he says with attention. "You're a writer, I'm told, but a seer as well. I'll have to introduce you to Major White who fancies that sort of thing. He's persuaded by unseen forces he refers to as metaphysical."

"I will look forward to that. I have a crystal even," Daniel amuses.

"Perhaps you could help with my memoirs when all this is over, or my obituary. Kindly hand me my towel and robe."

Daniel stands and reaches as Sherman stands, then steps out and dries off.

"Destiny is calling you General. How will you answer that letter?"

Sherman quickly puts on the robe and ties it around his waist, still pondering the solution, "I shall have an answer in the morning but I first need to send a wire."

They walk out together into the hallway. As they part, Sherman turns to Daniel then Charles, who has been waiting, "My officers will be attending a late breakfast or early lunch with me. Have all of your guests and staff there as well, for I have a special announcement to read. Good night."

He turns and retires to his room.

Charles, with his usual unquestioning response, answers crisply, "Yes, General. Good night sir." He pauses quizzically, "Which does he mean, Mr. Daniel sir?"

"It's called brunch, Charles, brunch. Late breakfast, early lunch... get it? I'll inform Marcus what to serve."

"Brunch?" obviously perplexed, "Yes sir."

Charles leaves while Daniel pulls out Lincoln's letter and the envelope and gleams in thought,
Yes sir. We both have a date with destiny.

Sarah's Nightmare

It's late evening in the master bedroom. Most are sleeping, as Daniel is seated at his desk by the window entering in his journal.

Daniel Journals:

Words come to mind like Day of Infamy, the longest day, a day in the life...whatever. Today has been...

An unfamiliar sound coming from down the hall distracts him to pause and listen. He goes back to writing. A sudden SHRIEK coming from a woman jolts him. He quickly jumps up, grabs his robe, and heads out into the hallway. Another SCREAM is heard. It's coming from Sarah's room. Daniel hurries, but not before Stillwater, wearing suspenders and under thermals, flies by with his gun drawn in anticipation.

Outside Sarah's quarters, Daniel arrives to her door and sees Stillwater looking in. Daniel moves past him and is deeply alarmed while wondering what has happened. Marcus is trying to console her by her bedside as she's hysterically crying.

The baby starts crying, then Marcus looks at Daniel shaking his head before explaining, "The nightmares."

Then looking back at the distraught maiden he's bonded too, "We'z here, Miss Sarah." He pats her pale hand, "Please don't fret."

Daniel assesses the situation, "Take the baby to Mabel."

"Yessuh." Marcus agreeably takes the baby away then Daniel takes Sarah in his arms and holds her, looking up at Stillwater he assures him, "We'll be all right Captain."

"I'll be up if you need me," he says as he turns to take leave. Just then two guards show up. "It's ok," he dismisses them. "You can go back to your post."

Sarah whispers faintly, "I thought they were here." Daniel gently strokes her hair and forehead.

"Who Sarah? Who's they?"

Sniffling she offers, "The raiders."

"It's okay," he reassures her, "These men won't hurt you."

"It's too late," she refutes adamantly, "They ravaged my body and vexed my soul."

Daniel closes his eyes in empathy. She collects herself and sits up just as Marcus peeks back in the room unobtrusively. He enters with a small basin of water, fresh towels and drinking water, then sets them down. He leaves watching her.

She gathers her memory with a deep, drawn out breath. "My servant and I had just arrived home late night from my stay with my husband in Vicksburg. He picked me up from the station." Sarah still shaken, mentally leaves Daniel's arms to vividly relive her story.

Sarah and her driver approach a large plantation she once called home. Her first concern is the whereabouts of her father. "I saw fire break out and men running out with arms full of valuables. I started to hide when suddenly I was grabbed from behind," she narrates.

A huge, nasty looking, rugged raider wraps his arms around her from behind.

She starts to scream, so he cuffs her mouth. Her cries go unnoticed in the chaos of violence. The fire is rapidly expanding while several men with torches continue lighting the area as if looking for something.

"What have we here?" She kicks and tries to free herself so he throws her to the ground and holds her down. An older man being dragged out of the house cries out. It's Sarah's father. A raider knocks him to the ground demanding, "Where's your money old man? Ain't gonna do you no good dead!"

Sarah's father looks over at her being roughly man-handled and shouts, "Sarah!" to no response other than grunts and rough, sinister laughter. "Leave her alone," he implores, "Let us go."

Marcus bursts out of the house to help Sarah's father. Several raiders overtake him as more slaves take off running. SHOTS ring out as two slaves go down. The flames are rapidly getting higher.

"Daddy!" Sarah screams.

The raider holding her father down looks over at her being manhandled "Ain't she a pretty thing? You can save her a lot of pain ...just tell us."

"Please, anything... just let her go." Sarah's father is pleading with the raiders, but it is useless. They drag him away behind the house as he's yelling in fear. Three SHOTS are fired! Then the raiders come back around the house. Sarah frees herself from her captive and makes a dash for her father.

"No Sarah! Run! Get away!" yells Marcus. One of the raiders strikes a blow to Marcus' head and then runs after her. Three of them grab her as she starts screaming at the sight of her father lying in a pool of blood.

"No! Daddy!" she lets out in agony.

"I'm daddy now. Time for bed." They start laughing hideously, dragging her off to the barn as she's kicking and screaming. Marcus, rather woozy, sees them pull her into the entry and tries to make his way toward the barn. While two raiders are holding her down, the original raider is undoing his pants. Two more start ripping her clothes off. She's screaming for her life.

"C'mon Red, take her," they cheer him on.

"Bastards!" she exclaims as they wear down her resistance.

Red stands over her, "That we are pretty lady."

Red goes to move in to violate her. Unexpectedly, Marcus is at the barn door but he's swiftly overtaken with brute force. They press his head to the ground smashing his face and eyes toward the violence. He can't move but he's just feet from Sarah getting savagely raped. He's left feeling horrified and helpless, as he goes in and out of consciousness.

"Help me," she sobs. "Help me, please."

Red gets off her, just as the next one lines up for a turn. The barn is filled with frenzied noises and smashing bottles of liquor while in the distance a blazing fire lights the sky.

Sarah, now shivering, narrates to Daniel, "I blacked out. I don't know for how long. I came to and another was about to get on me."

Without warning, the attacker keels over covered in blood. Marcus is standing there holding a bloody Bowie knife. He picks up Sarah and carries her out.

There's carnage everywhere. Bodies of raiders lie bloodied with unrecognizable faces.

"I was so weak... I saw their bodies, he went crazy on 'em."

Only a silhouette of the house fire lights the black sky in the distance. Marcus carries Sarah away like an angel emerging from Babylon's inferno. Away from the fire, Sarah's eyes open slightly. It's the last thing she sees of the only life she ever knew. Gone to ashes, like her soul ... she felt dead.

Daniel strokes her hair and wipes her last tear.

"When I came to was next mornin' in a slave shanty camp down by a river. I'd been washed and cleaned up, but I could still smell the stench. I wanted to die."

She starts breathing anxiously hard. Daniel holds her tight as she is shaking.

"I ran to the river and jumped in to kill myself...but for Marcus...God, the nightmares." She buries herself in Daniels chest and curls up into a fetal ball. He covers her with the quilt and holds her through the night.

Brunch with Sherman

Early morning light comes through the kitchen windows. It's bustling with activity. Marcus and the entire staff of servants are preparing multitudes of dishes to be served, unbeknownst to them, to the highest-ranking Generals and officers that would soon take part in the largest liberation of massive slavery since the founding of our country. General Sherman himself would be hailed by the freed blacks as 'Moses,' by the time he reached Savannah.

Daniel, dressed in white Edwardian shirt and black period pants, walks in expecting to deal with coordinating the affair, but instantly is relieved to find that all is in order, thanks to Marcus' innate ability to run a kitchen and manage staff. The multiple scents of food being cooked and prepared are enough to water the palette of any royalty. The aroma of coffee now gets his attention. William notices his entry and pours him a cup.

"Welcome to Spagos!" Daniel delights, with his eyes set on the steaming brew. William hands him a fresh cup of coffee with pride and a renewed self-worth on his face. "Obliged William, you read my mind. So, who had the presence of mind to set the dining area so elegantly, which I noted as I passed through this morning?" he teased, already knowing the answer.

Proudly, Charles muses with Daniel, "I did as much last night, sir. Seemed to be fitting thing to do in the quiet of the night when all are sleeping." He breaks a smile, "One must properly prepare for a 'Brunch' such as this."

Marcus looks at Charles rather peculiar as Daniel winks back. He slips into his old accent out of playful spite, "Time for Charles to fetch dat cornbread outta da oven."

Charles plays along correcting, "It's 'that out of,' Marcus. And 'the' - it's an article before a noun – 'the oven'."

Marcus stops and closes his eyes slightly perturbed, "That cornbread out of <u>the</u> oven. Now go on and fetch it."

"Good," Charles is satisfied for now, "We'll work on fetch later."

"Ah! So, you're the tutor?" Daniel surmises the situation, "Who better than a Brit to teach the King's English?"

"Thank you, sir. Also, I've taken the liberty to acquire one Barrister Forrester, a local thespian and who is also well acquainted with the proper reading material to begin our lessons."

"Very well. Can't wait to meet him."

Marcus points with new demand, "You let dat" he stops himself with frustration, "'that' cornbread burn, I'll skin yo' hide!"

Laughter fills the kitchen...

Meanwhile, in the front of the house, outside the time portal, a van with satellite dishes and antennas pulls up into Daniel's drive way. Emo gets out with his son, both with gear strapped on their backs used to detect magnetic fields and source field energy, holding wands in hand. The open side door reveals a main computerized machine with a large 60" screen for monitoring the data. Emo starts heading around the house getting readings, waving his detector.

Inside the manor, movement is stirring about with everyone seeming to know just what to do. Between the army and servants, Daniel feels everything is in control. A comfort he thought he had lost. He doesn't want to appear without a function and decides a bit of fresh air would do him well.

Daniel steps outside onto the veranda and sees the Union army setting up across the creek. A wagon of blacks, from a nearby shanty village, ride down the trail pulled by a mule with their life's belongings. One aristocratic couple are casually strolling when unexpectedly, he sees a character way out of place, with odd equipment, waving a wand that's emitting buzzing noises. It's Emo! Daniel sets down his coffee and trots past the guard and approaches with excitement, "You made it!"

Emo, oblivious to portal human activity, is also elated. "Your readings are off the chart!"

"You see no one?" Daniel asks with anticipation.

"No, but you do, is that it?" Emo concludes from experience.

Daniel almost laughs. "This is crazy."

Emo holds the wand up to Daniel. The guard is watching Daniel appear to be talking to someone. Emo asks him to turn full circle as he measures his energy wave length. The guard now wonders about Daniel.

"Not crazy to me. I find answer. You are same wave length. Your heart. Traumatic shock," Emo conveys his deduction.

Daniel is anxious to understand. "My heart? Yes, when my mother died. I still have the arrhythmia chart."

Professor Emo explains, "Please, get me your chart. A human heart normally projects an electromagnetic field within a frequency range of eight feet. Any extreme emotions are usually corrected in short time. Not yours - stuck. I'm guessing the same wave length as this time portal I'm reading. That's why only you see. You also on a major vortex!"

The guard now calls over another guard for confirmation. "Are you watching this?" He looks at Daniel conversing to apparently no one.

"That's spooky," responds the second guard.

Daniel hurries inside then comes back out with his EKG chart and hands it to Professor Emo.

Emo is ecstatic as he compares the portal electromagnetic wave lengths to those of Daniel's heart. "They exact! Wave lengths are perfectly parallel. That's why you see this dimension in time. Why 1864, maybe because of vortex history?"

Daniel is now animating his arms. "Okay, I get that. So, are they real? I'm so emotionally involved with these people."

"You ask questions to right man. Emo is here. Have theory," Emo is bursting with confidence.

His son comes around the corner shouting, "Pop! These readings are whacko! I mean off the chart sick!"

Emo slightly startled and apologetic adds, "My son. My assistant. Datsuki. Means great helper. Most time."

He holds out his hand and shakes Daniel's, correcting his father, "DJ Saki. Wow! Cool duds! Halloween? Ha ha. You see dead people. Ha ha. Just kidding."

The guards are now both chuckling at Daniel. "This is getting' good."

"My son also music DJ," Emo reluctantly admits.

"Nice to meet you," Daniel greets politely.

Emo's device, strapped to his side, rings. "Hello?" Because of the solar cell interruptions NASA provided Emo with a military grade two-way phone system, not available to the public. Having an advantage of range and clarity, Emo decided to have each floor provided with one for emergency and security reasons. He holds the two-way phone to Daniel. "For you, that nut job, Professor Brandy. Aka Blow hard." Emo and his son both laugh.

Daniel, thinking it's a cell phone call, and still unsure of what time dimension he is being governed by, declines. "That's no use to me here. Tell him Sherman's arrived and get his rear end over here."

Emo responds in to the two-way, "He say you big ass. Get over here."

"I heard, you pissant," Brandy yells on the other end. "I'm on my way!"

Daniel's eyes widen as Emo hangs up. "But wait! I could hear him! How does that work?"

Emo talks in a Mandarin dialect and confers with his son. He turns to Daniel, "He is in your present time, like me. Weird, huh? We agree, items from past can materialize now. Future to past - reverse time, not so much. Your situation unique, we figure out for you."

Daniel looks back at the manor and remembers his brunch engagement. "Well, nice meeting you, DJ Saki. I'd invite you both in for breakfast but there's no Sushi. Ha Ha." Father and son both look at each other with pause, then laugh. Daniel turns and walks by the guards. "Carry on gentlemen," as he enters the manor.

One guard snickers, "That is one crazy son bitch."

In the library, General Sherman is conferring with a group of his highest command, conceiving a bold plan to march through Georgia to the sea. Those in attendance will command more than 60,000 Union troops and bring the South to its knees : Major General Henry Slocum; Major General Oliver Howard; Brigadier General H. Hudson Kilpatrick, U.S. Cavalry Captain O.M. Poe, Chief Engineer and Topographer. Poe is laying out maps upon a large table and one sergeant is handling the telegraphing.

General Sherman reads from a telegram.

Taken rebel seaport, Mobile Bay, have been secured and evacuated by the enemy, you no longer need concern. Your other plans to take Macon or Savannah can now be considered.

At your service, General Ulysses S. Grant.

"Gentleman, this is excellent news," the General confirms heartily.

General Slocum agrees, "Indeed, it is. What about Hood and his whereabouts?"

"That's our last unknown," Sherman says with an irritating tone." What he does might just determine our next move. Confound it! I need that confirmation from General Thomas. Damn, he's what we need to contain Hood in Tennessee. I know he can do it, why doesn't he?"

"Hood seems unhinged at this point," Slocum answers. "I've heard stories gathered from prisoners."

Slocum, sensitive to Sherman's earlier bout with depression and mental health, stops from calling Hood a mad man, which some believe to be true. He's stopped obeying Jeff Davis' orders (the President of the Confederate States), while Confederate generals to Sherman's east are guessing where Tecumseh will attack next. Rebel desertion is high and reserves and militia are hardly formidable. Others have retreated to Alabama, expecting Sherman to march there. Observably so, the entire South is confused and in complete disarray at this point. Between military leaders, politicians, and Governor Brown of Georgia, the right hand doesn't know what the left hand is doing. That was part of Sherman's brilliance. Keep the enemy guessing with small decoy's the general would send out, like bread crumbs to send the enemy on a rabbit trail of erroneous information. These false mind games are what finally allowed Sherman to conquer the rest of the South in four months. Grant soon followed after the fall of Sherman's hammer, to tighten the noose around Lee to surrender, who'd been helplessly under siege for the entire winter.

"Leave that scoundrel to me," Kilpatrick bragged, "We'll chase him down like a rabid coon dog."

Laughter breaks out. Then Sherman wisely decides, "I believe that is exactly what he wants, to distract us from our mission. That is why I, with haste, backtracked from chasing his bunch into Tennessee. Waste of time. I'm awaiting a wire from General Thomas convincing, or should I say, a response from him, that he has the confidence with the 15,000 troops that he can assuredly hold Hood in Tennessee, which I affirmed him he could."

Howard, supportive of Sherman's strategy adds, "Yes. It would've greatly afforded the enemy advantage for them to have us to defend several fronts instead of our one - Georgia! And, perhaps return and take it. Good move Billy."

Sherman changes the subject, "Gentleman, I'm starving. We can continue our strategy after we partake of what fills the air like a scent from heaven's kitchen."

They all mumble and agree.

Sherman quietly tells his telegrapher, "Don't hesitate to interrupt me…everything's urgent now."

"Yes sir," replies the reliable sergeant. Sherman has set up a temporary telegraph station wired to the estate. Daniel will become not only acquainted with the telegraph sergeant but fascinated by its use and essential need for winning the war.

Sherman then grab's Cavalry General Kilpatrick after the last have left the room. "Have one of your Colonels immediately evacuate Atlanta of all citizens. Those are my direct orders. We can't take chances with rebel shenanigans."

"As you wish."

Daniel enters the parlor while Boone has readied his velvet-trimmed Edwardian morning coat and change of neck scarf. "How do I look?"

"Likes a peacock in a hen yad 'suh."

Marcus pokes his head in, "They're waiting on you Mr. Daniel." Marcus stands by the doorway in high-end servant's attire.

"Coming, Marcus. I must say you look debonair."

"I hope that's good, suh."

"It is, now y'all go on. I'll be there shortly." After they depart Daniel can't help but criticize himself *Ya'wl? My word, I'm in need of a tutor.*

The guests are gathering around as Daniel views from above the top of the foyer stairway. He notices Sarah mingling and moves quickly back down the hallway to her quarters. He sees Sarah's ribbon-tied letters and rifles through them. He opens the one with her husband's locket of hair and takes a few loose strands, then grabs a sample of her hair from a brush and puts it in another envelope. He quietly stands by the baby basinet with a sleeping Claire and stares at her innocence. *Now that I know your mother's mystery surrounding your time of conception, I would be remiss to not at least try and solve this ache in her heart. For you, I shall pursue the answer to this mystery.*

Claire opens her eyes and smiles. Daniel is warmed. "You're a sweet gift of a child... she loves you dearly." He relishes this unfamiliar, rare moment, then takes a swath of the baby's saliva with a Q-tip and places it in a glass jar. He hears a commotion from down below the slightly opened window. He looks out his frontal acreage and sees Brandy has showed up and is talking to Emo.

Brandy, in his mocking manner boldly bellows, "How 'bout aliens? Yeah, they'll be here any day now. You MIT lab rat. That's it. You're a failed experiment. HA!"

Emo is getting flustered and steams, "You head so big UFO land on top. Harvard is in dark ages. You behind times. Go back to school. Maybe this time learn how to bake cookies."

Brandy's hair is now standing at attention. "I'll take that wand and shove it up..."

Daniel appears, "Brandy. I'm glad you are here." The feisty historian settles down. Emo starts back toward the creek. "Wait professor." He pulls out envelopes and the glass jar from baby Claire's sample. "I need a DNA test run."

"For you, okay, maybe a week."

Brandy now ribs Daniel, "So, what's this about Sherman? You having a stroke?"

Daniel smiles, then turns and catches the guards snickering. Turning back to Brandy, he confidently does his best gruff voice, "Tecumseh, yes sir, Tecumseh himself." Daniel pulls out the Lincoln letter addressed to Sherman and Brandy carefully examines it.

Laughing, he bursts out, "Is this some kind of joke?" Brandy takes out an eye piece looking closely at the letter. 'My my, where did you get this?"

He hands him another letter adding, "I snuck this one out of the general's desk pile. He started a letter to his wife last night."

"Are you in The Twilight Zone?" He continues to examine, then questions further, "How did you know his wife was ill with child? That is, if you're supposed to be in 1864, that wasn't public until after the war. She lost the baby." He looks at Daniel with a 'gotcha' expression. He reviews it with more scrutiny this time and less skeptical.

"I've never heard of this letter. But that is his hand for sure and this ink is fresh... you're good."

Emo observes the situation and informs him thoughtfully, "I have theory."

"You have thewy," imitates Brandy.

"Communication getting through, unlike objects. Hair also old but hair is hair. I have idea. Things of same or similar material get through like letter, it's physics of Source Field."

"I'm confused," Brandy scratches his head. "There have been some strange stories coming from these solar storms, but I'll need better proof."

"You two figure it out. I have an early banquet to attend."

Inside the elaborate dining room, most are seated, with Sherman at the head of the table, then Stillwater arrives and seats himself next to the general. Daniel walks in and is seated by Charles at the other end near Sarah

"Ah, there's our host. The food has been blessed...shall we?" suggests Sherman.

They start serving themselves food as the servants pour cold liquids. Marcus sets down a second plate of bacon, knowing the first would quickly disappear. An array of eggs, bacon, chicken, potatoes, squash, melons and fruit are displayed in an inviting manor. A special plate of fresh bread, pastries and a dish of sweets prepared by Marcus also fill the table as a lively morning conversation begins.

Sarah fawns, 'Why Marcus, you have brought me closer to home than I ever could've imagined. Seeing this... daddy and momma..." Daniel holds out his hand to her. The others pause in respect. She tears, "It's a good thing. I'm not saddened, it's a fondness. Thank you all, please continue."

General Slocum validates her emotional response, "We share your fond feelings, Miss Sarah, as we miss so dearly our families as well as they miss their brave young men, we are certain. It is our intent to quickly remedy this misfortune, our nation truly mourns."

"Well-spoken Henry," Sherman raises a toast. "To our families, near and far, God bring us together swiftly." They toast and mumble in agreement.

"And, to our fellow commander, General James McPherson, whom you grieved more than anyone Billy, may he rest in peace," Slocum offers.

Sherman mourns, "Thank you kind sir, he fell before he could witness the final triumphant victory just days before Hood's retreat. A shame, as he was instrumental in their submission."

"*McPherson's death was a great loss to me*" he would later write in his memoir, "*I depended much on him.*"

After they were near finishing the food, Sherman stands to make an important announcement. "I have here an official proclamation by Secretary Steward from President Lincoln, establishing Thanksgiving as a Federal holiday." He looks at the memo again. "Indicating that it is to be the last Thursday of November." He looks at his fellow officers and chuckles, "When Grant and I finally agree upon a strategy, of which I am waiting his wire of approval this day, why hell, I intend to be halfway to the Atlantic by then with 60,000 men paving the way, eating off the tables of gallantry."

More agreeable chuckles, as everyone continues to feast on the lavish brunch spread, and the words of a leader they each admire.

Stillwater leans toward Sarah, "Nothing personal ma'am; it's war."

"None taken, Captain. I'm not attached to this God-forsaken geography. If you'll excuse me, I must attend to

Claire. Mabel, if you'd kindly bring up a plate of food and join me…gentlemen…"

Stillwater stands and pulls out her chair. She whispers in Daniel's ear, "You being there last night meant so much to me."

With chivalry, they all stand as she leaves the room, while Daniel absorbs her whisper of appreciation.

Sherman commands them to return to the affair at hand. "Be seated. It is my wish to celebrate as described by our President, Thanksgiving, only at an earlier date, say in two days, that is, if our fine host agrees?"

Daniel agrees, "Early Thanksgiving. Why not?" *A hundred and fifty years early* he muses to himself.

"Splendid. Stillwater, you arrange the hunting party for the appropriate game. Gentleman, I'll summon you to the library as soon as I hear from Grant." Just then, coincidently, the telegrapher hands him what appears to be three telegrams.

They all depart separate ways. Daniel intends to find Emo and Brandy when Sherman calls him aside. "I have your answer," he says, glancing at the telegram he is holding.

"Yes?"

Sherman reads it. "All or nothing."

"That's it?" questions Daniel.

"They refuse to release the black soldiers, or "their property," as they so word it. This is the major reason for the halt of prisoner exchanges, which we have amicably obliged during the war. They will only release the whites…Lincoln and Grant have stuck to their principle - all or nothing. I'm sorry sir." He then begins to light the telegram. "This also contains a confirmation…"

As the paper memo begins to smoke, Daniel reaches for it and pleads, "Sir, please, for posterity sake!"

Sherman shakes it to squelch the flame, without taking his eyes off of Daniel and smiles, "I was hoping you'd protest." As it smokes and the flame have died off, Daniel looks puzzled as Sherman hands it to him. "I need a biographer who can write with conviction." He places his hat over his high forehead and pulls it slightly down. "Excuse me, I have a war to win." He exits with two of his generals.

Daniel is left perplexed and deeply burdened. Sherman had also expressed he's been relieved of the mission to find the VIP and all focus must be on victory, and to conquer Georgia now. He leaves Daniel to contemplate the incomprehensible reason that 13,000 men had to die at Andersonville. Brandy was right, but Daniel got the confirmation straight from the source - Abraham Lincoln, General Grant, and General Sherman. Daniel takes the fire-singed copy of the official wire Sherman left with him and reads the words he referred to, *"March forward with courage and our blessing." This should be immortalized* concludes Daniel.

He invites Brandy, who is unseen by the guards, to come inside the manor. The guards look at each other and start wagering about Daniel's chances.

Daniel shows Brandy the charred telegram. Brandy's look is of amazement. "This telegram was only legend. It was destroyed or missing."

Daniel smiles and smugly asks, "I kept him from doing just that. Is that proof enough?"

"As close to convinced as I'm going to get," Brandy answers. "May I keep this?"

"It's yours, my friend. Welcome to my world."

Daniel and Brandy walk through the foyer and look around.

Brandy marvels, "What the hell? Your house looks like you could use a maid." He only sees the current condition of Daniel's house.

Daniel points out Sherman reading, as they pass by the library, "There he is." Sherman is in the library reading maps. "Come on," Daniels encourages the pace, as they proceed to the inner library.

Brandy shakes his head. "This is so not me."

"General Sherman, sir..." interrupts Daniel.

Brandy's look at Daniel is priceless.

Sherman looks up, "What is it my fine host?"

Daniel takes a pen and writing paper from the desk and puts it down for Sherman. "Could you please write a quick memo, noting the supplies I'm requesting for Thanksgiving are your orders?"

He takes the quill pen. "Why certainly, I do this every day. To whom do I address?"

Daniel keeps from cracking up. "The supply store owner is Mr. Langley."

Sherman writes, "I appreciate your hosting my officers. Are we in supply of ample amount of liquor? My men will be so heartened if so...it's our only solace during such times as these." "Liquor? Not to worry. I have a cellar full. And Marcus, my chef, is organizing a hunting party. Turkey, pheasant, and perhaps deer will be the bounty for the table. He'll make a great guide for Captain Stillwater."

Sherman and Brandy talk almost over each other.

"What are you talking about? This is bizarre."

Sherman replies, "Ah, I would love to join you. I'm constrained to strategy and logistics."

Daniel notices maps of battle plans, troop movements and various pins in place as he takes the letter.

"What's he doing now?" Brandy asks in amazement.

Daniel motions Brandy with a nod of his head, "Let's Go."

"Thank you, sir."

Daniel and Brandy are both giddy out on the veranda as he holds up the memo. "I can read it, can you?" Emo was right. The writing appeared legible to Brandy. "Tecumseh! A letter to me! This is nuts, but I believe it."

Daniel is relieved. "He's prepping for the campaign through Georgia to the sea."

Brandy is obviously envious. "You saw that? What's he look like? I mean, like his pictures? How does he talk? This is awesome."

They step down into the yard area.

"I'll fill you in. He was planning a special raid on Andersonville, for a VIP – a high-ranking leader, but canceled it."

"He's already had one failed attempt at Andersonville."

"It's in the letter...someone close to Lincoln. Family, he said." Daniel hands Brandy back the letter. "Also, earlier I heard something about expecting a raid on Sugar Hill. A spy informed him."

Brandy looks up the hill on Daniels property, suspiciously. "I'll study it. Meanwhile, you have got to persuade him to not engage in that battle. It was a senseless slaughter. It could've been avoided."

"Alter the course of history?"

They both stand there in awe of this prospect.

Daniel admits, *Knowing the future gave me a sense of power, almost godlike.*

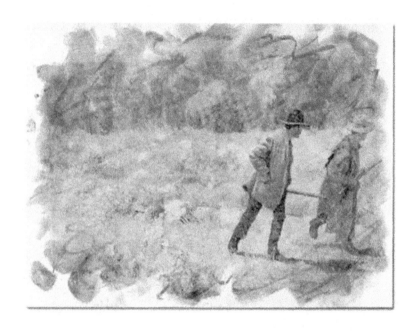

The Hunting

A new sunrise paints a beautiful hue as the plantation manor rises above a steamy fog that layers the ground. Morning light barely peeks through the forest, revealing an encampment of Union soldiers across the creek with some movement stirring about. Coming from the stables, Marcus is the first up gathering equipment for the hunt. Gunny sacks to carry dead fowl, ammunition horns for dry powder, and knives for gutting and carving on the field if necessary. Captain Stillwater walks out on the veranda putting a coat over his dressed-down look, armed with two rifles and a revolver. He didn't want to chance wearing his uniform as some Southerner might take a pot shot at a Yankee officer. "A fine morning for a good hunt and the last one for our healthy dinner game, wouldn't you say Marcus?"

"Yessuh. I hear tell you Yankees can shoot a squirrel's eye nigh a hundred paces, suh."

"One of my sharp shooters will be joining us for such as you say, as well a lookout for any rebs."

Just then Daniel steps out with two cups of steaming coffee and hands one to Stillwater.

"Obliged, kind host."

Daniel forewarns of his lack of hunting skills. "I've shot a pheasant in my youth. If I am to have any luck, it will have to jump right out front of me and stand still."

Stillwater chuckles as a well-equipped, civilian dressed, Union soldier crosses the creek bridge. "You can use this scatter gun. Good for turkey. We'll take care of the rest," Stillwater suggests.

Jackson walks up with Boone pulling a dual team of horses in front of a wagon. They all begin loading the back and taking seats. Marcus joins Boone in the front seat and takes the reins. Jackson double checks the horses' gear then pats them on the snout. "We'll take the wagon to the edge of an ol' corn stalk field and walk from there. I know a special place from there, spect an hour total," Marcus says.

Jackson cautions, "Don't shoot from the wagon, lordee, these horses will never stop." He and Marcus nod their heads grinning in agreement. "Wish I could join Y'all but I'z got a lame mare to tend to." He strolls back to the barn as the sharp shooter walks up.

Stillwater introduces his companion. "Gentlemen, this here's Emit Rose, finest sharp shooter in Sherman's army. Emit... Mr. Daniel, our fine host, and his servants...and Oh, Marcus here is the finest cook in these parts and damn good with that Bowie knife." They greet and exchange nods then begin down the trail and disappear into the morning dew.

Daniel's Journal:

I took one look back as the majestic mansion drew smaller and my sense of adventure grew larger. Hunting for our Thanksgiving feast, the fresh scent of morning forest, all without the modern conveniences technology had afforded me. I felt so alive. I realized I had come full circle in acceptance of my newfound life as one born out of due time. One glaring observation was that basic human needs hadn't changed. The need to be free, to care for one

another, to gather together and fight for survival if
need be, and that evil is constantly challenging our
way of life. Now we are about to partake in one of
the oldest and most basic needs of all. To hunt and
gather food, break bread together, and give thanks.
Not just to each other but, as Lincoln would declare,
to our creator, whom I must admit, I've given little
thought to in my latter years of success. I am now
open for more lessons of wisdom from my teacher,
the portal, which I so fortuitously encountered in
my lifetime.

Suddenly, a hawk glides overhead as the sun breaks
through and colors the sky several majestic shades of light.
Down the trail, the wagon rolls over the path becoming
clearer ahead. Every turn now becomes a painting, a canvas
of Southern countryside. Farm houses, barns and fields
aplenty, bordered by tall pine forests disguising the next
horizon beyond the bend. A few slaves in the distant field
catch Daniel's eye.

Journal continued...

How would I feel in the pangs of poverty and end-
less sorrow tilling the fields? Knowing the lash of
a whip, my first born being sold to a faraway land?
Waking up and going to bed with the blandest of
food, looking into the eyes of my black child. I can
only experience what I've been given. I can only
imagine what I have not. Knowing the future as I
do is little comfort, for they shall not know...for gen-
erations to come, the sacrifice it will take and the
rivers of blood that will flow.

Time hasn't passed long when Marcus pulls the wagon into high brush under an oak tree to keep camouflaged.

"We walk from here," he announces.

He ties the horses and puts an oat feed bag under each. They gather their gear and arms then begin following Marcus through the harsh foliage.

"This won't last," he encourages the group. "Watch those thorns, they'll tear your skin up."

After a few minutes of struggling and grumbling, they break through an opening. There's a small marsh to the left, an unused farm field ahead, a forest of evergreen tall pines, and amber poplar trees to the right. Two deer suddenly leap and blend into the dense thicket.

Marcus whispers, "No matter, there's plenty of them around and won't hear us no more."

They load their guns. Stillwater hands Daniel the shotgun and smiles, "You just make sure you stay in front of me. It's bird you want, not a Yankee Captain." He waves Emit forward. "What say you?" he asks for his expert opinion.

Emit eyes the terrain. "I say yonder, that rock ledge be good ground to get a field a site,"

Stillwater waves him on then the four of them start slowly walking the field. The sun is up from behind them and warms the air. Marcus points ahead as they all stop in silence.

In a whisper, Marcus directs, "Keep your eyes that away. I hear them."

Daniel keeps looking and listening. "What? I don't hear anything."

Boone motions to stoop down. They all huddle together behind some brush. He begins making gobbling sounds. They wait. Nothing.

Stillwater is restless to get a trophy in his sights. "I want some real game. I'm heading into the trees... find me a buck. You three carry on here." He heads toward the thick pine quietly and disappears into the forest. Boone and Marcus both start gobbling again. Quiet stills the air.

Abruptly, some distinguishable noise interrupts in the distance. Boone gobbles again. More distant gobbling is heard, but closer than before. Black dots move through drooping old corn stalks. Marcus' eyes widen, holding his breath, while Daniel is frozen. Reddish color forms around the moving black forms. Now more noticeable gobbling, as they break slowly onto an open area, with distinct thick feathers, heads bobbing, walking cautiously they come in to full view. There are five of them. One flares his feathers. Boone and Marcus cock their rifles. Boone nods to Daniel so he cocks both barrels, not taking his eyes off the colorful flocked creatures. The turkeys seem embolden now out in the open. BOOM. Marcus fires and strikes. Feathers fly as one drops to the ground. As they instantly scatter, Boone fires, and then Daniel. Marcus grabs another rifle and tosses another to Boone. BOOM. BOOM. Daniel covers his ears at the shattering noise. Then they all stand, waiting for the smoke to clear. Marcus grins from ear to ear then starts running ahead. He arrives quickly and holds a large fat one up by its feet. Boone and Daniel head toward the kill.

"Yesuh, yesuh, we gonna feast on this here dinna," brags Marcus.

Two more lay dead nearby when unexpectedly, a third bird starts flopping to get away. Marcus drops the one in his hand and quickly throws his Bowie knife, dropping a squealing wild turkey to the ground.

Boone is elated. "Lordy wez got four biggins."

"Hee hee, sweet Jesus!" Marcus is doing a little jig and laughing raucously at their good fortune.

Daniel smiles and examines the game. A sudden gun-shot echoes from deep in the forest. They all look and see a few deer scattering every which way.

"Must be the Captain," Marcus figures out loud. "Let's load these on the wagon. He'll be along,"

Boone and Marcus put the turkeys in large gunny sacks and head toward the wagon. Daniel is curious. "I'll check on Stillwater." He walks toward the area where the shot rang out. A strange stillness now cautions him to slow his pace. He stops near the edge of the trees and shouts, "Captain Stillwater?"

Nothing. He takes a step, crunching leaves as a small branch cracks under foot. Out of a clearing about a hundred feet ahead, bursts forth an ugly black formation, heading full speed toward Daniel. He's immobilized with fear. *What to do?* It's now closer, moving faster and double in size. He hadn't reloaded his chambers. Unarmed, he braces for what's coming. Barreling toward him is a vicious wild boar with sharp tusks and angry eyes, snorting with rage. Daniel turns and runs screaming for Marcus' attention. He trips and the boar gains ever closer. He quickly recovers and stands up into a full bolt, as he knows he's running for his life. Marcus hears his cry in the distance and grabs a rifle, but he can't see that far. Hundreds of pounds of wild flesh are about to crush, mangle, and tear Daniel apart. He can't escape the danger and turns to face his fate just feet from what he thinks is his last breath. BOOM! The boar drops and quakes the ground beneath his feet. Daniel's heart is pounding out of his chest and he is breathing loudly. Marcus calls his name from a short distance behind him. Just then, Stillwater runs up with his revolver in hand and surveys the situation. "Are you hurt?"

Daniel stares intently at the beast, and then to Stillwater, while still huffing for breath. "My God! He's huge! … I owe you my life."

Stillwater grins then looks afar. "I didn't fire a shot… it was Emit." He bends down to examine the lifeless animal. "Deadliest shot I ever seen… stopped him cold right in the head. Damn! You are one lucky soul, Mr. Daniel sir."

Daniel turns and sees Emit waving his hat in the distance. He in turn waves his. Now quickly, he's overtaken with that arrhythmia chest pounding. Things start spinning around him and he grabs his heart. The elements of past, present, and future time are flashing around him. Marcus takes notice, "Oh Lordee, Massuh Daniel, you need to sit down a spell." He sits and within a few seconds everything is clear and back to portal time. "I'm fine now," he reassures everyone, as he takes a drink of water Marcus hands to him.

Stillwater puts his revolver away. "Well then… Marcus, start cuttin' him up for the feast. Meanwhile, Emit can help me retrieve that fine buck I snagged with one clean shot before all this ruckus and carry it to the wagon."

Daniel stands a bit aghast. "We're going to eat that fowl thing?"

Laughter breaks out.

"I'll cut a special tender piece just for you Massuh Daniel. Cook it right. You be in hog heaven. We should gather some wild mushrooms while we're here getting that buck." Marcus leads Daniel, Emit and Stillwater to the edge of the forest. Moist areas around logs and undergrowth reveal a variety of mushrooms. Stillwater bends over to pick a few.

Marcus warns him, "No suh, not those…poisonous, give you dizzy spells. These here." Pointing to a damp patch, "Good for cookin."

They gather mushrooms for cooking. Daniel tastes one. "That might work with a good meat sauce." Stillwater sneaks a few of the poisonous variety.

Marcus, joking at Daniel's expense, "Yessuh, like a good, fat hog's meat."

More laughter. BOOM. A shot is fired from the wagon area. Stillwater and Emit bolt in that direction. In no time, they both arrive to find Boone holding two rifles, one aimed in the direction of three Confederates, the other still smoking from the barrel. Stillwater draws his revolver while Emit stops to take aim.

"Well, what have we here?" Stillwater goes into military Captain mode.

"I caught dem! Dez tryin' to steal dem turkeys. I fired in da air."

The Confederates stand still with hands high and unarmed with a rifle lying on the ground nearby. They look worn, scraggly, and with torn rags for clothing but for one, who still is slightly uniformed in officer stripes. Another soldier's head is bandaged with an arm wrapped in dried blood stains. He steps forward slightly. "We haven't eaten' for days... no ammo. We're done fightin'. Please accept our surrender."

Daniel and Marcus appear as Captain Stillwater takes aim with revolver on his sleeve. Daniel surveys the situation, and then recognizes the officer as the one first encamped behind his house going over maps.

"We don't take thieves and rebel spies as prisoners. We shoot 'em on site. Step aside Boone," commands Stillwater.

Everyone looks astonished. Stillwater cocks his pistol causing one rebel to back off. "Don't even think of runnin, my sharp shooter never misses."

Daniel steps forward and speaks to the officer. "I remember you. You gave me the dead soldier's belongings to give to his mother. What happened to your men?"

He now vaguely recollects also, then sighs and almost lowers his head. He looks at Stillwater, then back at Daniel. "Wiped out. All of 'em, 'ceptin maybe a few wounded left for dead in the fields or taken prisoner. Yanks swarmed around us like hornets."

The other rebel pleas, "Wez ain't spies, just dead tired a losin' all we know..."

Daniel moves closer to Stillwater and in a low voice to his ear suggests, "We've had a good day's hunt. Presenting these men to Sherman could only add to your stature...an added prize of sorts. Perhaps they could reveal of your enemy's plans or whereabouts. It would be a shame to leave them here behind, dead with nothing to show."

Stillwater stares for a moment then uncocks and lowers his gun. "Give em some water then tie em up. Let's load up the wagon."

Late that afternoon, returning down the trail, Boone and Marcus lead the horses seated with a wagon loaded with four turkeys, a cut-up boar and one large buck. Also, piles of sweet potatoes and corn from foraging the abandoned farm field and a basket of wild mushrooms picked at the forest's edge. Daniel, Stillwater, and Emit are seated facing back toward three confederates with hands tied to the wagon, walking from behind. Daniel contemplates their fate as he watches their engraved faces marred with war, suffering and survival. He breaks his silence during the other two's bragging of past battles. "So, Captain, tell me, what's it like killing a man?"

He hesitates briefly then answers. "That question should more resemble, what's it like killing your *first* man? Now that one... that's the one that leaves you feeling shattered to the core of one's soul. Then the mind does what it does best and starts rationalizing to suppress such feelings in order to survive. A cold deadness sets in. They become no longer men, but traitors. Objects that are hell-bent on destroying the Union... they just happen to bleed."

A small group of Union soldiers march by in single file alongside the trail making their occupied, conquering presence more obvious and motivating the Captain to add a deeper substance to his answer. Many were bandaged, limping, and wounded.

Stillwater sighs, "I earned these stripes on the battlefield, unlike some from military academies. The answer to which you are seeking Mr. Daniel is, 'Was it hard?' to which I say to you sir, what *is* hard and wearisome is watching those around you fall and die. Having them serve beside you, knowing their lives, their hopes, their loved ones...it questions life itself. To avoid such, I've found that undiminished and absolute detachment from God and man has become of necessity. I now only serve my country, its President, and the commanding General."

He looks out upon the countryside. A wagon full of Negroes, with piled belongings passing by gives each man pause. "Perhaps after this war I shall revisit God's place with man, but for now, complete and utter annihilation of the enemy with full submission is all I know."

The wagon comes to a full stop. More Union troops are crossing the road. Daniel looks back on the worn prisoners. *They know not what they're dying for. The fate of all mankind is always in the hands of the few.*

He steps down and takes the opportunity to give the rebel captives some water. As they start forward, Daniel decides to walk behind also. With only a half mile to his century period home, it all seemed like a long day's journey into odyssey.

Sarah's Dilemma

Sarah is pacing with child in arm on the veranda, looking out down the trail then back at her baby again. There is some activity involving the military across the creek and unfamiliar sojourners passing by... she is not paying attention to any of it. Her floor length dress seemed perfect wear for the crisp fall that set in since morning, yet exposing her bare feet with shoes flipped to the side for better pacing. Mabel steps out, wiping her hands with flour on her stained apron, concerned for the dear girl's state of mind. She decides to take a guess as to what is troubling her. "Miss Sarah, Marcus be along soon. Come inside and rest some."

Sarah turns and keeps the same pace. "Marcus doesn't worry me. He can always fend for himself"

Mabel takes another guess. "Chile you gonna wear that floor down frettin' yo mind over that Yankee Captain. Those young men in these parts been gone so long."

Sarah glances at Mabel, then back down the trail. "Just what do you suppose could be their delay just for a few turkeys? Besides, I've no mind for a soldier's safety."

Mabel walks out closer to her to peek at the baby as Sarah looks out again. "Daniel left his coat and gloves," she folds her arms in the slight chill of a setting sun. "A sure cold coming after dark."

Mabel now hears her true concern and reaches for the child. "I best take her now."

Sarah hands her over gently then with folded arms, takes a deep sigh. "Supposing they were to come upon a gang of those unruly rebels? They'd have no regard for his life."

Mabel now steps in front of Sarah and looks into her eyes. "Miss Sarah, I knew yuz fond for Mr. Daniel, but carryin on such...well, I sense some tender feelings goins on."

Sarah breaks the eye contact and turns looking out. "Whatever such thing could you be suggesting? He's old enough to be my father." She then turns back to Mabel with an earnest expression, obviously a noticeable change. "But he is of handsome quality, is he not?"

"I can't say bout white man's looks. I'm not used to such a question."

"Well, can you see he is charming? So well mannered, and he does have a way with words, makes him seem younger, but wiser too."

"We best sit-down Miss Sarah. Sometime a young girl just needs to talk a bit...quite a bit."

Inside the library, Sherman has gathered this, his final and formal meeting, with the core of his most trusted and formidable colleagues to unveil a strategy to slay the Southern Dragon with a blow to the heart of their infrastructure. The genius plan to destroy things instead of chasing armies and accumulating more senseless casualties was fine-tuned by the timeline of events and communication that led up to its implementation. The basic, unique, military element was to develop two major paralleled wings that made it almost impossible to penetrate.

Sherman was addressing another secret weapon, the pontoon trains that would enable his army to cross several rivers and creeks by the wagon loads, assigned to Captain

Poe, his chief engineer. "If we succeed bridging these crossings with the speed and ease which I anticipate, the enemy shall not catch up to our plans. Can I count on this feat being achieved, Captain Poe?"

"I'm confident General" as Poe points to areas on the maps "they will not anticipate us crossing these difficult areas, especially here in these waters that are not fortified with bridges. We must assume that several will be destroyed ahead of our march, as they will assume it will cause a major delay in our conquests."

"Conquests. Did you here that gentlemen?" Sherman looks around at his attending generals with a gleam in his eye then grabs his glass of Brandy with one hand and puts his other on the shoulder of his genius Captain. "A toast to our illustrious Captain Poe, whose maps and mobile pontoons shall enable us to tell stories to our grandchildren, while sitting by a comfortable fire, of the many conquests our brave army have waiting for us in the coming days ahead."

"Cheers." They all agree and continue formulating the strategy with which Sherman has given them the needed assurance to succeed.

Outside on the veranda porch, Mabel is holding the sleeping baby. Sarah has calmed down enough to sort out that she is much better off than just a few days ago. She imagines having a home but fears of losing it all again loom within her. "The comfort and style an older man can provide is attractive to a woman of any age, is it not Miss Mabel?"

"Got to be the right man... he can bring hell and fury too. Lordee, dez some crazy folk out dere."

Sarah, imagining her future, ponders aloud, "Sitting by a fire, comforted by his presence, his knowledge of books and art, not to mention perhaps a greater knowledge of the female anatomy, as much concern for her pleasure. Am I being too blunt, Miss Mabel?

"You beins too dreamy...theys can get lazy and bam, it's over and anotha chile on da way."

They both laugh. Mabel looks at the baby. "You can always replace a man, but you can't replace a chile. No siree."

When they hear the wagon approaching, Sarah steps off the veranda to greet them. She sees the wagon loaded but is slightly startled at the rebel prisoners and Daniel walking from behind.

Stillwater notices her concern and immediately calms her, "Miss Sarah, not to worry, they're secure. We've had a fine day of hunting, right Marcus?"

Sarah then walks up to Daniel and takes his hand alongside as the wagon continues toward the meat house. "How is it possible to fret over a man such, one I've only known a few days?"

Daniel is rather surprised but warmed by her revealing complement. "After all you've been through, how do you feel anything at all? But I'm flattered just the same," he responds.

"Your length of absence has caused all kinds of dreadful thoughts."

Marcus reminds her what's to come. "You forget all them thoughts when I'm cookin' these fixins, Miss Sarah."

Jackson greets them and takes the team of horses. They proceed to properly place the game in the meat house. Daniel moves to go inside the manor, as he's a bit chilled.

Stillwater sees an opportunity. "Miss Sarah, I was hoping, perhaps we could continue our conversation. I could fill you in on the day's hunt and Daniel's escape from near death of a wild beast."

"Perhaps," she says with an unsure tone.

"Good then. I'll change and join you later on the balcony."

Sarah starts to walk up to the veranda when Stillwater grabs her arm and turns her toward him. Boldly, he stares her in the eyes and conveys his true intentions. "I thought of you - returning to find you just as you are this moment... so beautiful, in need of a man's company to comfort you through this troubling period in your young life."

She pauses and looks into his eyes. Then, without responding, turns as he watches her go up the stairs. "Sarah." She turns back toward him. "You won't regret this."

Mabel looks at them awkwardly and escorts Sarah and the baby inside.

"Did you hear that?" Sarah quizzes Mabel, as if Stillwater was invisible. "I just knew Daniel was in harm's way. Never doubt a woman's feelings."

"Yes, Miss Sarah, yo's sho did know."

Daniel is turning in earlier than usual. Wearing a robe, with a pen and a glass of Brandy, he sits at his desk with thoughts he wanted to put into words before retiring, not chancing losing the feeling behind the words by morning.

Sarah is seated at her vanity brushing her hair. She stands to notice herself, then turns about looking in the mirror. No reflection can bring her justice. The fine strokes of Europe's most accomplished artist would struggle to capture her; a poet's living work. Charles knocks on her door. "Yes," she calmly accepts.

Charles enters and delivers her a note. "From the Captain, Miss Sarah."

She takes the note and opens it as Charles stands by. She then promptly sets it down. "Oh, just tell him I'm tending to a fussing baby."

"Yes ma'am."

He turns toward the door to leave. She primps a bit more as he walks away. "Charles..."

He turns toward her, "Yes ma'am?"

"Tell him I'll join him shortly."

He nods and walks out. She stops to reflect, then notices the letters from her husband, neatly stacked and tied by a ribbon. She holds them next to her bosom and tries to capture some semblance of a fragrance.

Overlooking the balcony, Stillwater is admiring the encampment activity across the creek. He sips from a glass of liquor then turns to find Sarah standing just behind him.

"The chill seems to have gone," she says to break the silence. "The night air is quite agreeable."

"I'd say so, now that you are here," he looks at her approvingly. "Can I offer you a drink?"

"Nothing strong," she returns. "A wine will do. Rumor has it you'll be marching out soon."

Stillwater is a bit surprised as he pours. "Even I know little of such orders. How is it you assume…"

"My sources, plus my instinct. Your Generals have referred to the Thanksgiving feast as their last here."

He hands her a glass of wine then stands close to her. "All the more reason to make this night special between us. I might not see you again…at least, under such perfect circumstances."

"Perfect circumstances?" she asks.

"Yes, you being alone and unspoken for. There'll be a lot of men vying for your affections after this war is over. Right now, it's just one man alone with you."

He pulls her closer for a kiss. She doesn't resist and closes her eyes to try and pretend it's her husband. A man in Union uniform, tall and before her at this vulnerable moment is all too hard to resist. He stops momentarily to look at her then sees she's open for another kiss with embrace, and is quick to respond. He's more aggressive this time; she feels more obliged than desirous of him. He runs his hands along the curve of her breasts and she pushes him back. He doesn't let go as she turns her head away from his lips. "I'm sorry Captain, please…" She has to forcefully stop him with a light shove of her hands and quickly steps back.

"We can find a more private setting," he blindly suggests.

"I was merely allowing a soldier a final kiss before he departs. My affections are not warmed beyond that. Please accept my apologies if your expectations were more than mine."

Stillwater grabs her again, as if he is entitled. "I will not be made a fool. You will learn not to resist further." Before he can pull her to a darker area inside, she throws the wine in his face and he releases her.

"The chill seems to have returned. Goodnight Captain!"

He watches as she departs, leaving him drenched and wiping his face with the back of his hand.

Daniel Journals:

I must confess, today has been quite exhilarating for life without cell phones, instant news or traveling by car. I've always envied men of the survival type; I'm not even handy with a hammer. To blend with nature, who will ensure you a day's meal. If skilled in the art of the kill, to pursue until the final conquest, you and family will be rewarded, fed and fulfilled. This communion of odd fellows, with one common goal, to survive, is the ultimate dance of survival and reward. I can now add a turkey to my venture into the wild, opposed to aisle four at a Walmart meat section.

As for the countryside and its populace, intriguing in scope of variety, that is - skin color, rich and poor, soldier, deserter, wounded or those tended to by nurturing women, who themselves are torn apart by grief for son or husband. This generation carries on what most would consider a constant struggle, no time to ponder such fancy notions as a driven purpose in life or what's trending with technology. I really wonder how fair it is to be born in what particular time in history is best suited for that person. How would Marcus fair as a restaurant franchise owner and remain humble and loyal, one who would kill to survive? Stillwater, his world view might have a chance at a more peaceful resolution had evil not dared him to become the same in order to defeat it. These prisoners in chains, what is their crime? Picking up a gun against a perceived invader all over the misguided elitists who fear losing their fortunes and power by enslaving those that are less than animals? I'm sure if I asked any of the three, 'were they slave owners?' what their answer would be. It is the night before, and I am now most curious to see how the course of events, which have brought this strange group together in the middle of the most divisive time in our country's history, will unfold and be played out on this Thanksgiving Day celebration of 1864.

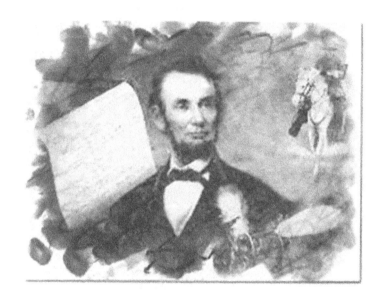

Amazing Grace, how sweet the sound, Through many dangers, toils and snares

T'was grace that brought us safe thus far, And, grace will lead us home...

Thanksgiving, God and Country

DINING ROOM – AFTERNOON

The table is laid out with the game from the hunt, with the exception of the boar's head, upon Daniel's insistence, well-seasoned and charred to perfection. The side dishes of potatoes, yams, and dressing, are surrounded with vegetables and complemented, once again, with specially created dishes in fine Louisiana style that only Marcus' secret recipes could provide. Who else could get away with crawdaddy stew on such an occasion? The setting is impeccable, a meal fitting a king before conquest, and also a gathering of grace and gratitude amongst those about to be seated.

William T. Sherman is standing at the head with his generals and their officers all in full dress uniform. Sarah, in a beautiful gown, is already seated with a center flower arrangement before her. All the servants are standing behind chairs waiting to seat the guests. Daniel walks to the other head of the table. There are three empty chairs with settings placed in front of them.

Daniel clears his throat "Gentleman."

'Nods and sirs' are returned. They're seated as Sherman remains standing. "I have here an official declaration by Secretary Steward from President Lincoln establishing Thanksgiving as a Federal holiday." He looks at the proclamation again. "The declaration indicates that it is to be the last Thursday of November." He then looks at his fellow officers with glee, now holding up a wire and continues confidently, "Grant and I have finally agreed upon a strategy. If not for the stubborn pride of a few for the lost cause of the many, this would be a feast of celebration. Never the less, we will hand them the defeat they so deserve." He sets the wire down then proceeds to the Thanksgiving Proclamation. "In any event, it is my wish to celebrate this honorable occasion right here at this time…giving thanks and honor to our founders, our God and country, which at this hour is so deeply divided with the agony of war and the weeping of women and children. I'll ask Mr. Coffee, our gracious host, to do us the honor of reading from this, our first official declared federal holiday from our President and our chief, Abraham Lincoln."

Daniel stands, a bit taken by surprise. Sherman hands the official letter of proclamation to an officer who passes it to Daniel. He can't believe the document he is holding.

Sherman motions, "Sergeant, you can bring in our other guests."

He signals and the three captive Confederates walk in bearing chained cuffs, yet wearing full uniform taken from other prisoners. The sergeant removes the cuffs and they are seated at the table. Daniel notices a show of some curious expression among the others. "Gentlemen, General Sherman, guests, and our staff, please come around closer."

The staff gathers around as Mabel is patting the baby. Daniel begins. "It has pleased Almighty God to prolong our national life another year, defending us with His guardian care against unfriendly designs from abroad and vouchsafing to us in His mercy many…"

The rebel's faces are finally looking up.

"…and signal victories over the enemy, who is of our own household. It has also pleased our Heavenly Father to favor, as well our citizens in their homes, as our soldiers in their camps and our sailors on the rivers and seas, with unusual health. He has largely augmented our free population by emancipation…"

Daniel looks up at Marcus. A few of the slaves start shaking and tearing up. They know what emancipation means more than anyone.

"…and by immigration, while He has opened to us new sources of wealth and has crowned the labor of our workingmen in every department of industry with abundant rewards. Moreover, He has been pleased to animate and inspire our minds and hearts with fortitude, courage, and resolution sufficient for the great trial of civil war into which we have been brought by our adherence as a nation…"

Mabel hands the baby to Marcus.

"…to the cause of freedom and humanity, and to afford to us reasonable hopes of an ultimate and happy deliverance from all our dangers and afflictions:"

Mabel drops to the floor and wails through her sobs. The other servants are mumbling prayers under their breath. The rebels are looking down, hiding their watering eyes.

"Now, therefore, I, Abraham Lincoln, President of the United States, do hereby appoint and set apart the last Thursday in November next as a day which I desire to be observed by all my fellow-citizens, wherever they may then be, as a day of thanksgiving and praise to Almighty God, the beneficent Creator and Ruler of the Universe."

Sarah wipes her tears. Daniel's hands are shaking.

"And I do further recommend to my fellow-citizens aforesaid that on that occasion they do reverently humble themselves... (now, slightly choking up) ...in the dust and from thence offer up penitent and fervent prayers and supplications to the Great Disposer of Events for a return of the inestimable blessings of peace, union, and harmony throughout the land which it has pleased Him to assign as a dwelling place for ourselves and for our posterity throughout all generations."

Daniel pauses here and looks up and around the room. No one is without an emotional expression of tiresome pain, humbleness, or thankfulness in tears of grieving forgiveness.

"In testimony, whereof I have hereunto set my hand and caused the seal of the United States to be affixed." Daniel sighs and completes the reading. "Done at the city of Washington, this 20th day of October, A.D. 1864, and of the Independence of the United States the eighty-ninth." He concludes, "Signed... Abraham Lincoln."

Sherman gathers his composure. "That was well done and quite moving. Thank you, Mr. Coffee. Let us eat what God has provided us...and be most thankful for the hands that prepared it."

Daniel nods and the servants begin serving. Mabel adjusts the baby and works with one hand. Daniel observes her strain and takes Claire and puts her on his lap.

Sarah takes notice and looks at Daniel with esteemed admiration. "Why Mr. Daniel, you sure would make a fine daddy. Oh yes, a husband too. When you read those words of Abraham Lincoln, my soul was so lifted like a dove taking flight. Such freedom in every word. You truly have a commanding voice and delivered it with such authority."

Daniel blushes, once again surprised by her unfiltered honesty, as the other officers look upon her with envious eyes. He has come to now realize and appreciate that her unbridled openness, blended with such affection, is an attractive characteristic, even surpassing her beauty.

Sherman, acutely aware of their distraction, reminds them, "Gentlemen, please, pass the food... I have a Brandy and cigar waiting for me."

Some laughter warms the room.

Daniel, seeking to be fed more than just food, quietly turns, "Sarah, you really felt that?"

"Mmmm," Sarah agrees with her mouth full.

She was right. He felt those words flowing through his veins; having read from the pen of the highest in command, before those entrusted to win this war and to those whom this war is being fought. A victory so needed by our country, orchestrated by God, according to the President's faith, *and here I stood, the only one in the room who knew the future outcome of the war - and the final fate of Abraham Lincoln. It was an honor I never could've imagined and a feeling I will never forget.*

Sarah spoons potatoes into Claire's mouth. "There, sweetie. Daniel look! Baby Claire took her first bite."

Daniel comes out of his thought and experiences another feeling he'd never felt before - the love of an innocent baby in his care. How could this be? A lifelong fear was gone. The fear that having a child would make him feel old or burdened. He was experiencing just the opposite now. He scooped up a spoon of pudding. "Let's try something sweet baby Claire," glancing at Sarah, he reassures, "girls do fancy the sweets." She takes the pudding in her mouth and gives a cute wiggle of delight. Sarah starts laughing and the others join in. "And they fancy being spoiled and getting attention, don't they Claire?" her mother coos to her.

Daniel was having an epiphany, a breakthrough, as was everyone smiling and enjoying the festive occasion. They were all a family. For one joyous, splendid moment in time the portal had removed all barriers and superstitious beliefs and given them a glimpse of heaven. To God be the glory on this Thanksgiving Day. It was a sight to behold.

Ironically, having earlier read from Lincoln the plea for peace and restoration to a divided people and a broken land, Sherman held in his hand the confirmation that such language had fallen on deaf ears, and knew what he had to do. As he led his two Major Generals into the library, he read from an earlier wire he'd requested sent directly to Jefferson Davis, Governor Brown of Georgia and Robert E. Lee, with permission from Grant. A final offer to surrender and also leave Georgia unharmed. Under the current situation, the South was hanging on the edge of annihilation. They had no chance of succeeding. Sherman's foresight was merely a formality he thought, in order to save lives the greater entreaty. After reading the short but emphatic reply of no intention of surrender, Sherman lit the paper of the prideful fools on fire!

"Gentleman, Georgia Will Howl!"

General William Tecumseh Sherman left in the dark of night, yet it was a darker night in the soul of the South. Death was coming to an aristocracy that had arisen, despite that our founders had deplored such a tyranny and left behind in Europe. A new dawn was coming for the black man and woman, a Constitutional freedom they had originally intended for all. Unbeknownst to Sherman, he would be hailed as Moses by the massive following of freed slaves on his march to the sea. He left to an undisclosed site north of Atlanta to wait upon the only factor remaining between his forces and victory that was not in his control – the weather. Those officers inside the manor had also left to various strategic locations. Stillwater and his Battalion were just over the hill waiting for orders. The soldiers encamped across the creek were in the process of pulling out as Daniel watched from his veranda. *It was a remarkable site to behold* he thought, knowing that in approximately 60 days they would be a part of 60,000 troops who marched on foot 285 miles. The South had no chance. The only thing left to defeat was their morale.

Alter the Past

S pread out beyond the creek on Daniel's property to the West was a sloping valley that rose up to meet the top of Sugar Hill. Daniel is up early riding in a carriage approaching a small Union camp that had been established since departing his lower property. Brandy had informed Daniel that history had shown the Union's plan was to draw the last remaining regiment of Confederates nearby to defeat them in an easily outnumbered battle. However, hundreds of deaths on both sides resulted from the senseless battle. Had the Union simply ignored them upon moving out, hundreds of deaths would've been prevented as those Confederate's would've proved inconsequential to Sherman's plans. Brandy's plan was to convince Major White to withdraw a day sooner and save his men from such a misfortune.

Daniel gives a confident nod as the guards recognize him and let him pass. He notices one young blonde boy dressed in uniform and folding the flag. Daniel walks up to him, a bit surprised at his age. "Hello there. You do that very well."

"It's my honor to carry the battle flag," the young lad looks up humbly, "like my ancestor."

"Your ancestor?"

"Yes sir. Served under George Washington."

"You should be proud," he gives the lad a wink and asks, "You know where I can find Major White?"

Daniel hands him some chocolate then the flag boy escorts him to Major White who's in his tent.

"I'll tend to your horse and carriage," the lad offers.

"That would be fine."

As fate would have it, Stillwater is approaching on horseback and notices Daniel.

Inside, the Major is looking over maps. He looks up and recognizes Daniel from his short stay under Sherman. "Ah, Mr. Coffee."

"Major White."

What stood out to Daniel the first time they met was his slight limp, he assumed from the war, and his silver, curly locks extending almost to his shoulders. He never saw him without his worn looking hat on, even the night he found him lost, walking down the gallery hallway in his undergarments. He kept a stylish mustache and bearded chin and the only other time Daniel ran into him was in the library. He loved Daniel's book collection, which they discussed briefly. The Major picks up a note from the table and a copy of the historical battle that hasn't happened yet which Daniel hand prepared. "Billy mentioned you could see into the future. He was most impressed," he chuckles, "how much bigger could his head get when you said he was a legend?' They both have a laugh at Sherman's expense. "I've read your courier letter and this battle record. How in the devil can this be? Are you really..."

Daniel's imagination and fiction writing experience kick in. "Yes sir. I'm a seer." He now proceeds to imitate his psychic experience and sets the pyramid crystal he purchased on the table. Nearly the size of a small jewelry box, he uncovers it with a bit of flare. It's beautiful, as prisms of light pass through.

"Like Nostradamus," he remarks. Brandy had also provided Daniel with some background on the Major. "Fascinating. I too am a student of Occult Studies and the hidden mysteries. Why, even King David had his seer named Gad." He picks up a wild flower out of a makeshift vase and recites "To see a World in a Grain of Sand and a Heaven in a Wild Flower, hold Infinity in the palm of your hand, And eternity in an hour."

"William Blake," Daniel says with confidence.

"Yes indeed. Excellent. Please, have a seat. A shame we didn't have this time together during our short stay under your hospitality. Ah, but time is such a fleeting butterfly."

"Fleeting but visible, for I am able to see into its mysterious maze of events. With my crystal pyramid, it has become quite clear."

The Major is enthralled. He looks at Daniel's letter. "Fascinating! Please. You mentioned altering this battle... that it can be avoided. If this record is true, then you're suggesting that time and events can be altered?"

"That is the question I propose we test, for I've had a parallel vision, one with a more desirable outcome." Daniel stares into the crystal then asks for a personal item from the major. He hands him his scarf.

"Go on."

"In the past, I've merely given warning after given such a dire glimpse into the future. However, since it involves those I've come to know, I felt a greater need for confirmation. So, I asked the source again."

"Like putting out a fleece."

"Let me demonstrate my method." Daniel closes his eyes and holds his hands over the crystal, then feels the scarf next to his face. Stillwater, who's outside the tent, eases closer to listen in. "In my vision, I saw peace without loss of life." He opens his eyes. "This confirms it, for I have seen the same vision twice, that establishes it."

"That is a premonition I can live with." He realizes his response. "No pun intended." Now easily convinced, Major White wants the same. "I am not of this war, I am in it. I will avoid bloodshed at all costs. Tell me what to do."

Moments later, Stillwater departs, like Judas at the last supper.

Daniel boards his carriage and begins to head back down to the manor after having given Major White the plan Brandy suggested. The young lad shouts as he's departing. "Thank you, sir, I fed your horse." Daniel turns to see the lad proudly smiling. Daniel smiles back acknowledging his deed and heads back downward.

It's an unassuming open field sloping from a distance below to the top, with one exception- the wild flowers. Charles had informed him of a wealthy couple from England he once served, who had brought over an array of garden flora and herbs, not all native to America, and both exquisite and fragrant. They left as soon as the war broke out, leaving their garden to the wind and the wildlife. Charles told Daniel his property, and especially the small valley at the foot of the hill, was the beneficiary of their abandoned seed and not to miss it. While returning to the manor below, he stops to admire the beautiful sea of color above the green grass. He steps out of the carriage drawn closer to the blooms. Wandering through a meadow of Lavender flowers, he touches the petals of a few here and there, releasing a fragrance that stimulates a powerful déjà vu effect.

Daniel rapidly searches through his mind, as one does, to catch that illusive feeling of having experienced this before. At that moment, a stronger sense of a female presence is felt around him, in a soft and gentle manner. He can almost touch her. The wave of flowers causes him to stare into the midst until her form appears in the distance. She's holding a basket, collecting the Lavender blossoms and stems, her bonnet blocking the sun just above her neck-line. With her back toward Daniel he calls out to her, but no sound comes out of his voice. He wants so strongly to see her face, but she dissolves into the field, just as the shadow of a cloud passes over. When the warmth of the sun resumes, he looks up to see not a cloud in sight then back upon the empty floral meadow. *How uncanny. Perhaps I am a seer... for I did see 'heaven in a wildflower.'* He heads back to his carriage and orders his horse home, returning his thoughts to the present. *I must walk this field again. Maybe a picnic with Sarah and Claire would be nice.* He sees two deer grazing in the distance. Peering down on the manor, he wonders what magic the portal has in store for this night.

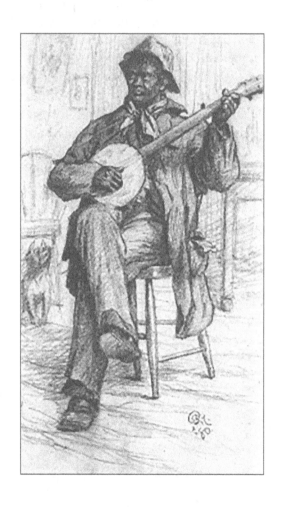

Dancing Miss Sarah

Daniel is fitting attire in front of a mirror listening to William play banjo while sitting in the corner of the master bedroom. Daniel glances at the reflection of the window behind him as it nears sunset.

Sarah is in her quarters getting helped with her dress by Mabel for this special occasion of the evening's festivities. Her hair is up and layered just enough to stay but loosely cascading strands down the middle of her back and sides in just the right places. Lace, silk and velvet drape her curves.

Out in the upper balcony the remaining servants are decorating by hanging lanterns, lighting candles, setting a table with flowers, wine, cheeses, bread, and a bounty of delicacies. Daniel has arranged a Victorian lounge sofa for later relaxing.

In the kitchen, Marcus is preparing desserts fit for a queen while singing, "Camp town ladies sing dis song, Doo-dah! Doo-dah!..." He puts the tasty morsels on a serving tray after one into his mouth and admires the presentation. "Oh, Miss Sarah gonna love this night. I know how to get to a woman's heart, yessuh." He leaves for the upstairs balcony with the tray.

As the servants continue their activities around the balcony, an elegantly dressed woman is rehearsing violin in a corner area just as Daniel enters like a peacock. She turns the music sheet in front of her oblivious to the activity around her. Marcus sets down the tray with a silver cover at a servant's station.

"Splendid. You're a saint, Marcus," complements Daniel.

Obviously, a joyous Marcus replies with a big beaming grin, "Mr. Daniel sir, sho fine idea to have this here to cheer up Miss Sarah. She's been lookin' for this all day."

William enters with his banjo, bows to the violinist and is seated next to her. Daniel samples the hors d'oeuvres. Marcus then leaves as the music tuning stops. Daniel turns at that moment and his heart speaks when he first sees Sarah. He would later write in his journal *as a songbird that approaches, just as the last glorious ray of sunlight plays upon her golden hair, highlighting her blue eyes and colorful wear. Enter the wind that lifts her perfume through the air.*

His eyes follow in an approving downward review of her long soft gown and warms a smile at her bare feet upon the ground. Anxious for his opinion, she moves closer. He is beholding a poem unfolding.

The banjo and violin come together and play in a sweet harmony. Daniel's thoughts are flowing but he's unable to speak. "I'm struggling for words to describe how I feel right now, and I'm a writer."

"You're the man of the hour, my knight. You came to my rescue."

"And you to mine," he returns with a deep gaze into her eyes.

Charles appears with apron over one arm and opens the wine and pours. Daniel and Sarah toast. Charles steps back by the doorway. "Here's to time standing still, this moment is forever ours."

"My, for a man with no words, you sure can take the breath out of me."

They set their glasses down and slowly dance, facing each other as the evening takes over.

Oh Dixie Bird I'm lost in your eyes
Yes I'm out on a limb
Twirling you in the wind
The trees are calling your name
Oh Dixie Bird your freedom cries
Oh Dixie Bird I know you must fly

They drink and sample the array of food. She bites into a piece of chocolate cake with delight then puts the remaining morsel in his mouth. He laughs then makes fun of her bare feet with a slight tickle. Sarah takes sips straight from the bottle then twirls so freely with a happy smile. The evening is splendid as it deepens into the night. After the servants have retired, a few hanging candle lanterns remain flickering... just the two of them sit, reaching for each other's hand, looking up at the stars.

The moon is out above your hair
Do I hold you and rock you?
Til you fall safely asleep
Or a kiss on the cheek do I dare
Oh Dixie Bird your freedom cries
Oh Dixie Bird I know you must fly

Sunrise dissolves the dark. Daniel is sleeping on the open lounge sofa sitting up. Sarah is lying in his lap with eyes closed while the baby sleeps next to Daniel to his other side. From a distance, a man in war torn Union uniform is slightly limping through the field of high grass. Sarah's eyes open slowly, seeing a distant figure. From the front, the soldier is walking like a man on a mission. Sarah sits up quickly, her eyes now fixed on him closing in. *Jonathan?* Her heart jumps her to her feet. He sees her coming toward him from the manor and tears begin dripping down his whiskered cheek. She's running to meet with him as he is limping faster. She flings her arms open and wraps them around his neck. "Jonathan!" she cries as they embrace and begin passionately kissing. Her father's watch falls to the ground as he madly twirls her in the air.

When morning broke I awoke
I could still feel you in my arms
You gave me something I can't explain
His love returned you let go of the pain
Oh Dixie Bird your freedom cries
Oh Dixie Bird I know you must fly

The baby dissolves away and disappears. Sarah is gone.

Daniel Journals:

In the Psalms, it says a thousand years in your eyes are like a day that has just gone by. Sarah was a song in the night for a thousand years. I never got to tell her that her husband was the baby's father. She has shown me that love is stronger than blood. They will be happy, somewhere in time.

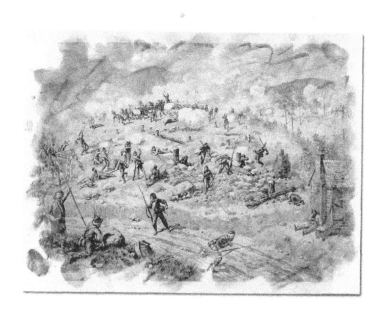

Covered in Blood

There seems to be more fall color in the landscape surrounding Daniel as he walks his property. Up much earlier than usual, he catches nature's activity in every direction at the slightest glance. Wild mushroom growing on deadwood, a woodpecker's early drill up above, a fox he's never seen disappears as quickly as he appeared. Squirrels that were once plentiful seem to have vanished, along with his favorite red Cardinal. What do they know? There's a time for every season - his mother's favorite saying from the Bible. To Daniel it was from a song he grew up with. *To everything (turn, turn, turn) There is a season (turn, turn, turn), and, a time to every purpose under heaven.* Daniel wonders what season he is in. The portal will soon reveal the coming change.

Jackson and Oakley pull a saddle horse out for Daniel and help him get on.

"You be all right?" asks a concerned Oakley.

"Riding a horse is like riding a bicycle. You never forget."

Daniel rides off to the Union encampment on top of Sugar Hill.

Oakley turns to Jackson, "What's a bicycle?"

Daniel rounds the forest to the great open valley toward the top of Sugar Hill when crashing EXPLOSIONS and distant SHOTS are fired – smoke billows everywhere! His horse rears high as Daniel holds on. He's is shocked at what he sees. It's a full-on battle charge! Cavalry, infantry, artillery, appearing from several directions, are on a collision to destroy. *No! This can't be happening!*

He races through the valley and heads for what appears to be the officer in command about to lead another wave of Union soldiers into the battle from the hill. Cannons are firing a barrage from both sides, some blowing up near Daniel's path. He reaches the commander. It's Stillwater.

Daniel cries out, "Why are you doing this? This wasn't the plan. Where's Major White?"

"I'm in charge now, Major Stillwater," pointing to his uniform, "and here's the plan: crush the enemy and take no prisoners. Now get out of my way."

Daniel looks back at the hundreds of men converging "This is mad. The war can be won without this bloodshed," he pleads.

"War is bloodshed and victory to the ones who carry out orders." He pulls out his saber to charge and stares down Daniel. "You and your likes stand in the way of victory," then shouts "To victory!"

The men shout "Victory!" A cannonball ROARS overhead and blows up Union ranks nearby. Daniel moves out of the way as they charge down the valley and witnesses them gun down a group of rebel artillery. He turns and pursues up the hill to the encampment of the officer's tent to find Major White lying deathly sick in a bed cot. No one is tending to him. A bowl of soup is next to his bed and some vomit on the ground.

Daniel is extremely upset. "Major. What's happened?"

The Major opens his eyes. "I feel dreadfully nauseous… I suspect…"

Daniel recognizes the poisonous mushrooms in the soup. "My God!"

"I can't say for positive..." he gags. "Stillwater convinced General Slocum when he got word of our plan."

"So, he gets promoted because you're deathly sick."

"It's a disaster."

"It's Shakespeare." Daniel looks out the tent at the mayhem and starts to leave for help.

"Mr. Coffee..."

Daniel turns to face the stricken old veteran soldier.

"What of your vision?" He strains to slightly lift up and gives a look of hopeless despair. "I believed in you."

Remorse renders Daniel speechless as the Major closes his eyes and lays back moaning in pain. "I'll get you help from below." As Daniel rides off into the valley, a cannon ball EXPLODES and throws him off his horse, causing him to black out.

It's nearing sunset of the longest day. What was once a field of splendor has become a ground soaked in blood. Daniel is lying amid dead, mangled corpses and wounded bodies, sounds of coughing and moaning through the lingering smoke. He raises up, then peeks his eyes open as he slowly stands, looking from one end to the other, aghast and sickened.

Scavenger hawks and ravens circle above the carnage. A few men are sauntering in the distance looking for wounded. Though Daniel is stunned, covered in black powder, and stained in other's blood, he has not suffered an injury that he can tell. He staggers from body to body in disbelief when he spots the flag. A feeling of horror fills his gut as he walks over and looks down, then dropping to his knees, he wearily lifts the flag to reveal the mangled face of the young lad. Daniel looks at him with such anguish before he buries his head next to his. A murky haze fills the air.

Daniel raises up, his face now covered in the young lad's blood - with a look of determination in his angry eyes on one goal. A fury has engulfed him. Daniel crosses the creek, appearing through the haze, carrying the dead boy under the flag past his manor on a mission.

Out of the portal, he's now turned and walking up the hill to his hip black neighbor's house. They are casually mingling outside in the back drinking and talking while J. J. is standing by an older man, his father. Daniel walks up to them with only the bloodied flag now remaining draped in his arms. The attention from everyone is now on him, having all come to a complete stop.

Daniel commandingly exclaims, "Raise the flag!"

J.J. confused at what he sees can only stammer, "Excuse me?"

"Raise the flag!" Daniel insists.

"What's he sayin' pop?"

His father gently attempts to take the flag, very carefully from a crazed looking man "I'll take care of this. Just chill," he assures carefully.

The iconic flag flying is hoisted down while the tattered and soiled American flag of 1864 is raised. It unfurls in a gust of glory.

Daniel Surrenders

The following morning in the countryside, Fitzgerald is parked at the gateway entrance to the historical plantation property she pitched to him over the phone. An obvious 'For Sale' sign is posted nearby, where she's standing by her car on a cell phone. "Well I know, dearie, but you're going to have to come down off that price a bit...I need some leverage. Oh, here he comes now."

Daniel pulls up as she gets in her car and he follows. They come to a grove of trees, with two standing fire places among a previous plantation ruin. There's a rustic old barn and another grove of orchard trees with a fragmented private cemetery in the distance. When they get out, Daniel looks tired. He obviously hasn't slept.

A cordial Miss Fitzgerald approaches not knowing what to expect, only she knew Daniel had called her unexpectedly with a renewed interest. He certainly didn't sound himself during their brief phone conversation. "That was the owner I was just with on the phone. She's willing to..."

Daniel sees a small house that appears to be in good shape, down the property road. "That's the furnished house with modern amenities?"

"Why, yes. Built ten years ago for..."

"I'll take it. When can I move in?"

She is wondering at Daniel with genuine concern "I'm sorry you had a falling out with your other home - just too many bad memories?" No response. He's staring at the barn. She sees a broken man. "Your mother I mean."

Daniel drifts back more coherently to the present moment. "You're probably right. I just want to move on and let it go."

"In all my years of doing this, trust me, I've seen it before and people do recover with a new beginning."

Daniel is now looking at the small cemetery of about five grave markers. "I don't suppose you can have those moved?"

"I'm not sure. It's a Southern thing with some legal issues. Will you be listing the other property?"

"Never mind, they can stay." Daniel starts to get in his car.

"Oh, I almost forgot," she said, attempting to get his attention a while longer, "Your agent called."

Daniel smiles, then gets into his car. Confused and bewildered, he's now wondering if he should just keep driving until he reaches the arms of his understanding wife. When he pulls up to his manor he sees Emo's van and Brandy's car. There's more gadgetry spread out on the lawn which Emo and his son are testing. As he gets out, Emo starts to say something when Brandy steps in between and gestures for him not to say anything.

"I got your message," Brandy starts. "My God, man, you must be devastated."

"I'm leaving," Daniel says sternly. "It's over. I've got to get out of here."

"Look, I know we...you just got kicked in the guts trying to play God..."

"They're lying in that field," he looks off painfully.

"I blame myself," Brandy confesses. "Who was I to think men's lives could be placed on a game board and moved around like some chess pieces? I'm new at this, too. We'll know better next time."

Daniel turns to Brandy and adamantly assures him, "There's not going to be a next time, Brandy. It's over."

Brandy looks back at Emo's anxious expression, then to Daniel, "You can't leave now. You're ancestor. If you run away now this will always haunt you. It's your heart and your past, you've got to reconcile this...this...deep pain inside you. Look, Emo...he's got this theory..."

Daniel looks at Emo and his son while making a hand gesture of frustration. "No more theories."

"...to get us all in," Brandy finishes.

Daniel stops and stills his gesturing. "What do you mean all of us?"

Brandy's eyes widen "You, me, and Emo. What do you say?" He pauses then enunciates, "Andersonville!" Brandy leaves the ball in Daniels court and lets him ponder, looking at the equipment, as Emo continues watching with anticipation. Daniel folds his arms and looks at them. "More hell and misery...this madness is folly. There's a full bottle up in my room...I plan on drinking all of it my last night. I'm finished." He walks off.

Later that evening, Daniel lies in bed staring at the ceiling with a half empty bottle. *I've lived long enough to learn that with everything that feels good, there's a tradeoff. I was feeling empowered, a return to my intuition- in sync. Then I woke up in the land of death. The dogs of war had won. Not a tradeoff worth going back in. I surrender. Finding my ancestor in Andersonville is off my plate. Getting back what I had with Michelle seems much more attractive to me now. I'll weave a quick story from my other house – hopefully, with full solitude. I'll tell Michele that it won't be long.*

His thoughts are calming down as he feels the booze and the release of surrender ...but underneath, something is still calling him. And he knows it will be there as soon as he awakes.

The Map

The following morning, a sluggish Daniel starts to gather his ancestor's letters and belongings when he smells breakfast. *What's to become of his servants? I'll miss these comforts and food.* Marcus' cooking is a special delight that stood out to Daniel. He did not dare look out his window at the view of the battlefield that once laid mild in such peace. *I'll pack, then eat, and be on my way with this feeling of fondness before it slips away into a cold, cynical self-pity.* He knew not to dwell, as if he were the responsible one, and had caused such a dreadful event. Nevertheless, he felt a belonging. It wasn't like him to leave anything unfinished, except when it came to himself. He was as good as a man was going to get, he thought. Flawed, selfish, but just maybe good enough to find one more story to flush out onto the bestseller list. *I'll think about it after coffee,* he assures himself.

Marcus is at the door and addresses him in excellent proper English, "Excuse me, master Daniel. Could I have a talk with you, sir?" Daniel is cautious, as he remembers the last calamity when he asked for a talk. But he decides to complement Marcus on one obvious note, "Your speech! It's working."

"He's a strict teacher, but made me understand that proper language is my future when this war is over."

"He's right. It will open a whole new world for you."

"That's what I came to talk to you about. Sir, I want to be free now."

"You've thought this through?"

"Well sir, now that Miss Sarah is gone and you're leaving with the soldiers out fighting, maybe the raiders will come back."

"I've thought of that, too." Daniel knows Sherman is about to turn Georgia upside down and the majority of slaves will revolt to freedom, but not everyone makes it.

"They will burn your house down and either kill us or sell us," Marcus reminds him.

"I agree. But not before you got in a few jabs yourself."

Marcus shyly smiles. "Too many of them. If we run from here they will eventually track us down. There is another way. You can sign a manumission declaration and pay our way to freedom. Then we head north." He pulls out what appears to be a tattered map out of his shirt then spreads it out on the desk as Daniel gets up and looks. "Before the raiders came we knew better, and Sarah's father had us bury his fortune here on the plantation grounds." Marcus points to the spot which is also detailed and circled. "We'd surly get caught trying to dig it up now. It's lawless. I'll give you this map and you buy our freedom." Marcus stands and looks at Daniel as a man. "It's a fortune, sir. It's yours. I just want to be a free man, raise a family and cook my way through life."

"What about Sarah?"

"She knows. She said she would never set foot on that ground again."

Daniel has the money to honor Marcus' request without the map, but realizes his pride is a primary virtue to him, so he accepts his offer.

"Well, what do I do?"

"Could we meet in the library? Marcus asks. "I'll have breakfast and your coffee served in there? "

Daniel enters the library to find a man dressed in a wig and 18th century Baroque attire. Daniel slightly confused looks around at the decor and realizes it's till 1864.

Marcus makes the introductions, "Our tutor, Barrister Forrester sir, this is Master Daniel Coffee."

They shake hands and make introductions, "I'm Daniel."

A proper Barrister replies with a British accent "Excuse my attire, but I also fancy myself an actor in between my legal duties and tutoring. A local play dress rehearsal, even in war..."

Daniel interrupts a bit playfully as if imitating a British accent, "*All the world's a stage, and all the men and women merely players.*"

Barrister is delighted. "Ah! *They have their exits and their entrances, and one man in his time plays many roles...* Shakespeare at his most insightful. Do you believe in his seven stages of man?"

"I'm beginning to believe that there are eight of them. And, I'm stuck there now.

"Marcus, I'll take my coffee. Tea or coffee, Barrister?"

Marcus waves Charles and William to begin serving. An array of fresh cooked food is laid out on a table already covered in a fine dining cloth. Charles hands Daniel his hot coffee.

"Tea for me thank you, however, I've already eaten ... oh, my," he grabs a pastry, "perhaps another time we can continue with that conversation." William pours him a tea with a saucer cup. "However, your slave here, Marcus, has asked me to write out a manumission for he and his fellow slaves, with your granting permission and payment in full, of course. I can return by morning with full documents in hand with proper signatures for each individual."

Daniel goes over to a safe hidden behind books. He returns with a leather pouch the size of a pillow. "What is the price of a man these days?"

Forrester pauses at the large bag of money. "Well stated Mr. Coffee. How we value life has come to how we view society and the world, hasn't it?"

Marcus is uncomfortable with the conversation, but his freedom is at stake along with his kin.

"$1200 should suffice the fine state of Georgia, plus a small fee, say, $200. I hope you understand by my doing this where my sympathies lie, Mr. Coffee."

"Why, in your pocket book, Barrister." He hands him the cash.

"Touché'. I've met my match. I shall return in the morning. Mr. Dupre, Mr. Coffee, good day."

Marcus shows him out and to the door.

Daniel starts up the stairs and feels someone watching. He turns and looks down. He sees a row of the whites of the eyes of all the slaves gathered. Mabel is smiling. Daniel is moved. *Perhaps this was my purpose.*

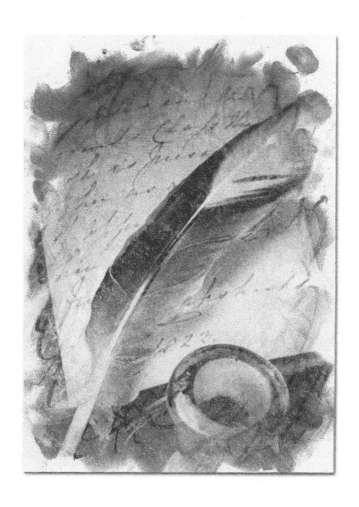

A Child is Coming

Later, while sitting at his writing desk, as Daniel prepares to leave, he resumes going through his family items when he picks up his mother's old Bible. A letter falls out, along with dried, fragrant lavender petals. *That fragrance again.* He notices it is a different hand writing than his great – great grandfather's, yet appears to be from the same period. He opens to read:

"My darling husband, may your path be brightened with His comfort and protection. Your call to duty most honorable, most valiant, has kept us safe at home and your country is most grateful for you and those brave men under your command. Beloved James, it's at this time I must tell you with ecstatic joy beyond my dreams that I am with child. Yes, it's true! A miracle night with you. Now father can no longer hold back his affections. Our last visit he feigned happiness at seeing me, he's so weary with the decisions of war on his shoulders. This child will bring us all a hope for a better future.

My, how the seasons change so swiftly here. I do hope you liked my poems. Mr. Whitman has been so

*kind with his attention to my prose. Here is the one
I wrote the moment I knew of our newborn to be."*

Daniel turns to the next page. It is in beautiful cursive style.

*Oh, unforgettable night, a coupling by fire
Brings new life, nature loins a young sire
I bare the joy in the aftermath
Keeping aware of any movement about
A new song I sing, as I follow the path
Light shines forth an array pure and sound
Colors now abound, but still
My heart shall not rest until my loved one is found
With cheerful face gazing into the precious eyes of the gift
of His will.*

*"I do hope you approve. I can't help feeling it's a
boy. My work at the infirmary is calling. I must go.
I dearly fawned over your last letter. God keep you
in safe hands.*

Your affectionate wife,
Rachel

Daniel is taken by this complete surprise. A love story
spoken so divinely before from the pen of her husband, but
now has been surpassed in poetic verse which compares
to the best of the romantics by his wife's literary voice
and composition. She mentions Walt Whitman. That must
be who she refers, of whom Daniel is familiar. He was
well moved to write of the times during the Civil War. She
mentions her father *"with decisions of war on his shoulders."* His mind is now thinking, *This is no ordinary wife,
or daughter,* which adds a cloud of mystery surrounding his

ancestor, or ancestors, both of whose statures have just elevated before his eyes. *This letter was hidden in my mother's Bible. Surely, she read it. This is a game changer. I'll give it more thought. I need a sign. Yes, I shall look for a sign. Either I abandon this fantasia or I pursue with the passion of a man on a clear path. I need the mission clarified. If the portal has the answer, then show me.*

Daniel had formerly planned a lunch with his Aunt Margret, after which they were going to lay flowers on his mother's grave. He wondered about telling her or even showing her Rachel's letter. Knowing she'd be thrilled, he brought it with him. She chose a local favorite spot with outdoor seating, as the weather was accommodating, plus her sister would occasionally meet her there and Margret wanted to share her memories with Daniel. She was the caretaking type personality so her concern for Daniel was greater than for herself. Hopefully, she could relieve some of his pain, although wise enough to know that grieving is a necessary process that everyone goes through in their own way. Daniel greets her at the front door with a kiss on the cheek. "You look well, Aunt Margret."

"Oh, you would say that no matter how I appeared, but thank you." Always colorfully dressed, she did take special care in her fashion, makeup and hair, as all three of the sisters had well into their seventies. He opens the door to her petite frame.

"This is a lovely place," remarks Daniel as he looks around the quaint surroundings with a rustic old farm theme. "I'm feeling right at home," he jokes to himself.

A hostess greets them and Margret requests a table outside. The air holds that crisp fall feel that most in the South look forward to, a relief from a hot, humid summer, hoping the comfort will last through the season. After both settled for a fresh salad, he struggled not to think about

Sugar Hill and chose to keep his focus with his Aunt. She was reminiscing about her dear sister and shared those stories from long ago… some of which he'd never heard and was delighted to listen about his mother. Aunties are great for that.

"Sometimes we'd get the giggles so much it hurt."

"Oh, how could I forget that?" Daniel recalled those laughs, too. "You two would wake me up at all hours when you came to visit."

"Your father threatened to send us both off on a long trip, bless his heart." She looks through her purse and pulls out a family picture when they were little girls and shows Daniel.

"The three of us were close, but your mom was my hero. Growing up in the Midwest in a small town…well, not much culture. She went off on her own to college, a big city girl then. But she always came back to see us sporting the latest hair style, and showing off her new fancy clothes. After momma and daddy went to bed, we'd stay up listening to her stories about city life…but all we wanted to know about was the boys," she laughs. Daniel notices her conversation has taken off some of the edge of his battlefield trauma. He hopes he can manage the graveyard visit without too much pain.

They drive separately a short distance to the cemetery. Aunt Margret pulls an arrangement of artificial flowers that will last through the coming winter until she can visit again in the spring. Daniel walks ahead of her for a private moment. As he arrives at her grave he's met with an unexpected site that freezes him still: lavender flowers, freshly bundled and tied together around the middle of the long stems with twine. *It's her! The mysterious girl in the lavender meadow.* Now the fragrance adds to his intoxication. He's transformed and feels her presence again. *This is it!*

The sign! He's sure of it. At this point he doesn't question the how or who, he's learned to just go with it.

"What is it Daniel?" Margret asks from behind.

"Someone has been kind enough to leave her some fresh lavender."

"My, aren't they beautiful? Oh, and that smell...they are fresh." She reaches for them and holds them close to her nose to enjoy the fragrance and affirm her intuition. "Yes, English lavender." She sets them upright, leaning the fresh bundle on the grave stone as she arranges hers. Daniel is now only thinking of one thing - getting back to the portal.

That evening, Daniel, now used to lantern lighting in his manor bedroom, finishes his drink. He takes the recently found letter and holds it next to his heart as he drifts into sleep. He slips into a dream, rarely a part of his night's rest. This one was vivid. His mother was sitting next to him packing his suitcase.

"You'll need a warm coat. I've also included some fruit for snack." He looks at her with concern. "Don't be afraid," she assures.

Daniel loses her vision but hears her voice clearly enough to be awakened, "Find Him."

Startled out of sleep, he quickly sits up. He'll contact Emo and Brandy first thing in the morning.

We're going in!

We're Going In!

D aniel didn't even have to contact them, they were parked creek side on his property when he woke up. Brandy is lying on a blanket wired to a machine while Datsuki is managing controls in the van. Emo looks like he's right out of the ER, holding a customized defibrillator with gloves. Daniel rushes downstairs and outside to greet them "What's going on?"

"I put settings to simulate shock, death, and trauma... his heart into like yours...wave length...you know what I try to say."

"Yeah, your theory, however, our dear historian here has to have a heart to induce arrhythmia," Daniel chides.

Brandy sits up. "If this whack job's thewy is right, well, if my heart gets on the same wave length as yours, I should see the time portal too."

Emo hands Daniel two gloves attached to wires. "Put these on."

"What? You want to fry me too?

"You won't feel a thing. Must line up electrical wave-length to yours. Remember I tell you? We must create the collective heart field, that's the key.

"Ok, I get it." Daniel puts on the gloves attached to Emo's invention.

Emo looks at his son as he nods an affirmative, indicating that he's ready. Brandy lays back down then Emo jump starts his chest causing Brandy to jerk. "Ouch! Just kidding, I'm OK."

Emo tries again. Brandy jerks harder and he sees the house change, then back again. "I saw it! Your house. Something happened!"

Emo gives a thumb up to Datsuki. "OK. Go for it."

"OK, Pops. Pump up the volume and mash it up."

Daniel recalls, "Roast duck coming up. I can't look."

Daniel turns his head as Emo shocks him again. Brandy jumps up quickly and looks around in amazement. He sees the portal activity. "I'm in! I'm in history heaven!" He starts twirling and looking about in amazement.

"Arrhythmia!" shouts Daniel, as he removes his gloves.

Emo folds his arms, "Now who's the whack job? Ha!"

"Pops! We did it! Brandy? Can you see us?"

"Of course, I can. And you're still a couple a geeks."

Emo smirks, "Remember...you still gotta come back, pinhead."

Daniel looks at Brandy and smiles, then happily hug each other. Brandy can't believe this is real. A small cavalry troop trots by while Daniel watches Brandy's expression.

"Believe it my friend. We're in the cradle of the Civil War."

Emo is wearing a Yankee hat and marching around in a giddy fashion, saluting everything. He would try it next.

Daniel Journals:

When Emo entered the portal, he was a kid in a candy factory. He did make one disturbing comment however, the energy will get lower, giving us a small window of time before the portal closes, requiring

*us to leave by tomorrow morning. Emo would have
to figure out a way to stay in communication with
Datsuki to monitor the energy levels. We met earlier
tonight to go over details. We agreed on only one
back pack apiece and we'll go by train, taking the
wagon to the station. The scientist and the historian
had their reasons for going in - Emo's need to discover and invent, Brandy's to witness Andersonville,
but as for me, to find my ancestor, and figure out a
way to convince him that I'm from the future. I'm
also excited about Brandy's latest idea we hatched
together as the evening wore down.*

Daniel falls into a sleep after having mapped everything
out in detail, but the portal had other plans.

Early morning, the servants are loading the wagon
carriage as Daniel steps on to the veranda while Marcus
is pacing.

"Relax. Tell me, where will you be going Marcus?"

"Charles has family in Pennsylvania. Is that a good place
to be? When this war is over, I'm going back to Louisiana."

"Pennsylvania, yes, just remember, Philadelphia chees-
esteak sandwich... you'll be a wealthy man."

Barrister Forrester appears alone in an open carriage
and pulls up next to the wagon.

"Sorry for the delay - bureaucrats." He steps down and
opens his satchel. "There now. These are all in order...
stamped, signed, and official documents of manumission
with right of travel papers." They all look at the documents in reverence. Marcus steps forward and takes his as
Barrister makes it official.

"Marquis De la Jacque Dupre, you are hereby declared
a free man."

Marcus looks into the clouds. "Lord a' mighty, you might not recognize me with my proper speech so Iz gonna say it da way I knows best..." He starts dancing and praising, "Sweet Jesus make room cuz Iz comin to the promise land... hallelujah, I say." Shouting at the top of his lungs "Glory Hallelujah!"

Daniel's feelings mount and they bid farewell. *I will never forget that last sight of jubilee watching Marcus jumping all the way down the trail.* The others hug and kiss Daniel and hop into their wagon. Forrester starts to leave when Daniel invites him inside. "Mr. Forrester, come inside, let's have that conversation. I have a proposition for such a gifted actor as yourself." Daniel bows and Forrester proceeds inside.

"I'm always open to a worthwhile proposition, sir."

With his arm around Forrester he asks, "Have you ever heard of Andersonville?"

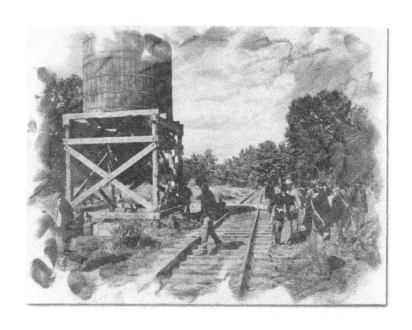

As news of the death camp reached the newspapers, Northerners were newly enraged at the South and its army upon hearing the miserable conditions and high death rate in the camp. "There are deeds, crimes that may be forgiven, but this is not among them." – Walt Whitman

Last Stop Andersonville

D aniel, Emo and Brandy are seated on the train with a diverse group of people boarding after them, mostly Southerners evacuating after the fall of Atlanta as Sherman has ordered the complete removal of all citizens. Some passengers are soldiers being transported, others are gamblers and vagabonds. Women and children are separated into one car. It was not your typical day at the train station. A dark cloud was moving in over Georgia that would forever change the land.

Daniel hands Brandy Rachel's letter he read the moment they get seated. "Read this. It doesn't sound like a letter to a Sergeant."

Brandy glances at the letter as he asks, "You sent the messages? In the order I told you?"

"I've been up all night going over our plan. I wired Captain Wirz via Sherman's telegrapher, like you said."

Daniel had been fascinated with the communication system during Sherman's visit, the telegraph wire. He had befriended one Sgt. Leonard and learned a great amount of this most fascinating invention from the 1840's that had revolutionized long distance correspondence. As the Sgt. displayed how to use the Morse code and its inventor's machine, he would tell Daniel stories of the exchanges between Sherman, Grant, President Lincoln, Horace Greeley at the New York Tribune, and a host of other well-known names that would sometimes come fast and furious in a steady stream, changing the course of battles and even political decisions. He even explained how they some-times sent the enemy false information, either directly, or knowing they were being intercepted. Intelligence decoys were used even back then, Daniel thought, since he had used modern methods in his novels.

Daniel remembers one time as they drank together, he let Daniel have a hand at sending a Morse code message... to the White House!

Mr. President – stop – You don't know me – stop – But it has been an honor to have hosted your fine General these few days – stop – a Union patriot, Daniel Coffee.

Daniel and Leonard laughed and drank together over that occasion. So, when Daniel sent a messenger to Sgt. Leonard the previous day for a special favor, he included a bottle of the Sergeant's favorite whiskey. Leonard had relocated north of Atlanta, where Sherman was waiting for the weather to clear to launch his famous March to the Sea.

Daniel recalls as he hands the young mail delivery rider a dispatch letter along with the liquor. "Now you take this and have my man do me a favor. Got it? Tell him specifi-cally the second one is to General Winder." General Winder, being the head of prisons in the region, and currently sta-tioned at Andersonville with a small regiment.

"Yes sir. I never fail a delivery."

After reflecting back, Daniel now turns to Brandy, "I made it sound urgent. Winder will be chasing his tail in circles."

Brandy chuckles at the thought of their plan working.

"So, what of the letter?" asks Daniel.

Emo leans over, "This is your great, great grandfather, yes?"

"Yes, that's from his wife. I know little about her. She sounds educated and writes poetry, it's all I know. Fascinating, her connection with Whitman who was in DC at the time volunteering at the medical hospital camp, is more than a coincidence. So perhaps she was there also at that time. However, my aunt mentioned her being in Missouri, not Washington."

"My, you've done some research," complements Brandy. "This reference to 'men under his command' is almost code, like she can't divulge his real rank. There's no address to his rank on the envelope, which is uncharacteristic. You're right, she sounds charming."

Brandy turns their attention, "Which reminds me, check these documents out. They match Lincoln's and Scranton's signature perfectly, with the U.S. Government seal." He compares letters Daniel obtained from Sherman with the documents he created. Gleefully he points out, "Photo Shop is a gift of the gods."

Emo can't resist. "No, MIT invention, but at least you good for something."

"Don't start in with that..."

"Once again, I find myself counting on your knowledge of history to pull off this plan," Daniel interjects.

"Trust me, this is going to work. When we do, it will become history. Recorded history! If there is a God, all powerful, all knowing, then he can go back in history and alter it for the betterment of mankind. Now that's what I call divine providence."

"Now I know, you sent from God. I did not know God from Harvard," Emo interjects.

Daniel kids, "Who knew a professor from Harvard believes in God?"

Suddenly the whole portal flashes like a quick short circuit revealing space and no environment, then back to 1864.

"Shit! What was that?" worries Brandy aloud.

A question that Daniel had never thought of before occurs to him, "What happens if we lose the portal Emo?"

Emo is looking at his meter. "Sudden drop. We lose portal, we stuck. Trapped for good in 1864."

Over the two- way Datsuki calls out, "You still there, pops? Better speed it up."

Daniel leans toward Brandy. "Ask God, what's plan B?"

Andersonville is merely a village in the afternoon, teaming with activity. When they step off the train the layout is similar as Daniel remembers from his visit. Brandy, who is anxiously anticipating what's around the corner, knows it even better. "This way," he calls for Daniel to follow.

"Prisoner morale suffered from the seemingly indifferent treatment of the dead. When a man died in the stockade, other prisoners appropriated whatever possessions he had not disposed of before expiring and often stripped the body of its clothes. They carried the body out to the deadhouse where corpses were kept, while awaiting transportation to the cemetery. The deadhouse was often already full; at times fifteen or twenty bodies or more had to be left on the ground outside it. Prisoners carried the corpses to the cemetery, and buried them without coffins in long, six- feet wide trenches."
– History of Andersonville Prison – by Ovid L. Futch

They strap on their rough back packs then mingle to look like commoners, and walk straight toward the prison stockade, just outside the village. When they round the corner, they're confronted with the horrifying sight and stunned at the sudden reality of corpses piled at the entrance to the prison. The smell of death is overwhelming as bodies are carried away right in front of them. Staff and prisoners have handkerchiefs around their heads with only their face-less eyes revealing.

There's a stack of what appears to be food, cornmeal and lard, with flies buzzing all over the goods in a nearby cart. Sharp shooters stand in the towers. There's a medical shack on the other side of the gate. A few limbs are in a pile with buzzing flies all around. The three are gagging and covering their nose and mouths, in complete silence, astonished at the gruesome sights.

Brandy chokes before he can cover his face with a scarf. "My God, no amount of books ever prepared me for this."

Professor Emo looks at Daniel with concern. "You still going in Daniel?"

"I've got to, I've got to know. Plus, I made a promise."

Suddenly a rebel Private walks up to them from behind with rifle semi pointed in their direction and calls out an order. "Halt!" They turn around and freeze. He quickly drops his role and confesses, "Pretty good, huh? I'm one of the team. The cast...you know."

The three of them overcome the trembling and sigh with relief, especially Daniel. "I'd say, pretty good."

"Scared the shit outta me," Brandy says with irritation. "What's your name?"

"Barrister calls me Shakespeare, cuz I love to act. C'mon, you're supposed to meet up at his room to change."

Daniel, Brandy, and Emo look at each other, then one more time at the prison stockade. Brandy asks Daniel a final time, "It's last chance, you can still change your mind."

"Last night when I read her letter, I heard her voice. I'm not sure I'm just doing this for myself anymore, something's calling me inside there."

"Then let the show begin."

They walk off and head into town.

The whole stockade reeked with an overpowering stench, and the men suffering from chronic diarrhea and others too sick to get to the latrines, deposited human wastes all over the stockade. An inspecting medical officer observed men urinating and evacuating their bowels at the very tent doors and around the little vessels in which they were cooking their food. Small pits, not more than a foot or two deep, nearly filled with soft offensive feces, were everywhere seen, and emitted under the hot sun a strong and disgusting odor.

"The condition of the stream, which was originally intended as the source of water for all the needs of the prisoners, was appalling. When the stream is swollen by rains, the lower portion of the bottom land is overflowed by a solution of excrement, which subsiding, and the surface exposed to the sun, produces a horrible stench." - History of Andersonville Prison- by Ovid L. Futch

ANDERSONVILLE STOCKADE PRISON - LATER

The gates open. Daniel, now in a Union Private uniform, is being led inside with dozens of other Union prisoners. They are stopped and the escorting soldier shows them in the gate as Daniel is thrust inside. They are immediately met by grunts (self-appointed directors), looking at his belongings. "Welcome to hell. You got any valuables they didn't get? Best hand 'em over and we'll take care of you."

Daniel doesn't speak, he just stares around at the volume of men, makeshift mini tents, and bustling activity.

"The sick and dying are yonder. No need to bed there. What outfit you with Private?"

"31st Illinois."

The grunt points. "That'd be Montgomery's men."

That's it! He's still alive, Daniel thinks with a silent victory.

"Just follow the creek till the bridge then turn right, there's a flag over his tent. You just see me, you need tobacco or whiskey. Cost ya, though. Blankets, shoes..."

Daniel walks off and is taken in by the faces of despair, loneliness, and sorrow. The aura of death is prevalent. They were all under fed, and a lot of skeletal figures with sunken eyes are barley clinging to life, obviously, wishing they were dead. Daniel approaches the bridge and turns down the row and sees the flag.

ANDESONVILLE TOWN- MAINSTREET

A confederate General is on horseback proudly heading down main street. He is escorted by two confederate soldiers. One is the Pvt. Shakespeare, who confronted them at their arrival and the other he is escorting, is none other than Barrister Forrester, dressed impeccably and playing the part of Confederate General Hampton. He has a long-waxed flip up mustache and goatee beard with authentic gloves, saber, and a feathered hat.

HEADQUARTERS PRISON CAPTAIN

There is a row of rebel soldiers standing at attention on either side of the stairway of this quaint wooden building. At the top of the stairway is a small man with a mustache and long gray coat. It's Captain Henry Wirz, the infamous warden, who was arguably burdened with the impossible management of a disastrous, poorly planned prison, and who would be later hanged for war crimes. Two soldiers step forward with the confederate flag and one with a Georgia flag. A Confederate officer sees the General approaching and draws his saber in salute fashion.

"Attention!"

The general and escort stop as the small man holds a salute. Captain Wirz properly addresses, "General Hampton, sir."

General Hampton responds with a refined, gentlemanly Southern accent. "Captain Wirz, I presume."

Captain Wirz steps down to greet him as he gets off his horse. They shake hands. "Yes General, we got your message. We've been waiting your arrival and have prepared for this..." he leans closer and whispers "...secret meeting of such importance."

"Excellent."

Captain Wirz gestures toward his headquarters.

STOCKADE

Inside the stockade prison, Daniel stands outside the Montgomery tent just staring. It's a real tent compared to the others. He finally gets the nerve and calls out "Sgt. Montgomery?" After no answer, he pulls back the flap and enters anyway. Intrigued by his belongings and every detail, he opens a leather-bound Army-issue Bible that is heavily worn, marked, and underlined. He touches his clothes and sheet then picks up a book of Dickens and thumbs through. He sees a few envelopes, a quill pen and paper, then picks up an open letter on top. It smells of the familiar lavender. When he opens to read, a chain trinket almost slips to the ground. He catches it and holds it in his hand while reading:

My fairest husband, at last I received your where-
abouts and am frightfully troubled. I notified father
as soon as I learned...

Daniel hears talking, sets down the letter and steps outside and sees two soldiers are being carried away.

"Here soldier, help with this."

Daniel turns and he's face-to-face with James A.
Montgomery. About thirty, handsome and younger looking
than he expected. He's about to help a soldier to the sick area
as he speaks with commanding English, "This man needs
our help, then we'll discuss why you're going through my
belongings."

Daniel snaps out of it and lifts the weak soldier as they
help walk him to a makeshift infirmary area. James questions while assuming, "You just arrived... don't drink from
the creek, stay away from those with a high fever, stay out
of the dead line and most of all, pray."

"The deadline?"

"The boundary line inside the fence where they shoot to
kill if you cross." Daniel looks up at the tower then remembers Brandy's description. "And they never miss."

They set the man down then James helps him get a drink
and makes sure a few others are tended to as well. Daniel
is now observing his every action and reaction. "You're not
sick? You look good, even better than your picture."

James stops, looks at Daniel as he pulls out his tintype
photograph. The look on James' face reflects his mind is
stirring. "Where did you get this? My wife, is she alright?"

Daniel now has to lay out every detail carefully. "I've
never met her, that was given to me by my mother."

"Washington send you?"

Daniel hands him one of his letters. "You have elegant
handwriting." Daniel studies his expression.

James looks around and back at the letter then pulls it out. "Step inside my tent." Once inside, James, baffled and suspicious, confronts Daniel, "Explain yourself."

"We're family. I'm Daniel... I'm a writer."

"Well, that's a relief. My wife's side no doubt. She's a writer as well."

"On my mother's side, she was a Montgomery. Your great-granddaughter...this is her birth certificate. You might want to sit down."

As they sit on the cot, Daniel pulls the certificate out along with a flat satchel stuffed in his pants and shirt with a specially made canteen of water.

"I do not recognize her name, and there's a mistake on the date. It should read 1835."

"No mistake. My mother was born 1935. I was born 1964. I'm here from the future, 150 years from now."

"But, my child is still in the womb. I'd say you were a madman yet I am fascinated. Do you write fiction?"

Daniel now looks surprised. "In fact, I do."

James pulls out a magazine with cover of science fiction stories. "Are you that science fiction writer, Sutter? He writes about time travel. I enjoy reading such fantasy tales."

Daniel examines.

"Yet, why are you choosing to write about my ancestry?" questions Montgomery.

Daniel shows him the remaining letters and James examines them thoroughly. Then has a look of deep awakening and concern. "There's nothing dated past this month and year." He looks up with a searching alarm. "Are you saying, I'm going to die in here?"

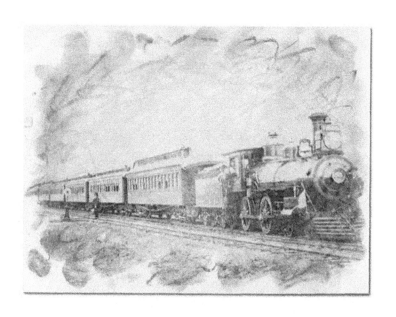

The Sting

HEADQUARTERS PRISON CAPTAIN

Wirz and Hampton are alone.

Hampton primes his ego. "Your cooperation and handling of this delicate situation will be duly noted in upper command. Your reputation here running this Yankee prison is quite legendary, indeed."

"Thank you. The train is on its way and should be here within the hour just as you requested."

"And it's passenger cars? Able to carry at least 2,000 men, correct? No, box cars?" Hampton confirms.

Wirz pulls out the paperwork and re-examines the details. "Yes, I've read you're orders and carried them out explicitly. This is not my first prisoner exchange."

"It is from Andersonville. Well then, let's make it official and get to the signing of this. We shan't keep the good Yankee General waiting any longer."

Wirz gestures, "Right this way, I've chosen the house of Madame Dunlap for this secret occasion. I assure you she is most discreet."

"Excellent."

They start out. "And, she stocks the finest Brandy and makes delicious cookies."

It's beginning the last stage of daylight as the sun begins to go down. The meeting house is only a few steps out the back where two rebel privates, one being Shakespeare, are on century duty at the door entrance as Wirz and Hampton step in.

DUNLAP HOME MEETING PLACE

They step in and see the back of a Union General viewing a painting on the wall. He immediately turns holding a glass of Brandy. It's William Tecumseh Sherman. Or, is it? Barrister meets Brandy for the second time and brilliantly play the roles they rehearsed the night before in Daniel's manor, with some lighthearted ad lib, of course. Brandy's 'Tecumseh' is in perfect form.

"Ah, there you are General. Forgive me but our gracious hostess has forced me to sample her vintage Brandy with such grace that I had to oblige."

There's some nervous laughter. Within the room is a single table with familiar fake documents spread out, a writing pen, three chairs, and a cigar box, with a candle and lantern. Wirz introduces one to the other.

"General William T. Sherman, this is General Hampton." They shake hands.

"T - as in Tecumseh. Fine meeting you again, General."

Wirz, a bit taken by his gruff voice, but more surprised at the comment. "You've met before?"

Hampton corroborates, "Under less fortunate circumstances, overlooking the battle of Chapel Hill, I believe."

"Perhaps less fortunate for you, as I remember it only took a couple of hours, for I had scheduled an opera for that evening," as Sherman might brag. Brandy grabs the bottle of liquor and opens the box of cigars. "Drink up gentleman and have a cigar, we're about to make history at this signing."

Wirz insists on formality and protocol, in spite of Sherman's comments. "If you pardon me, I still need to see your President's signature and go over it...and Scranton..."

Sherman looks at him with slight disdain, intimidating Wirz to lighten the atmosphere a bit "...that is for posterity...I feel honored to preside over this ceremony."

Brandy's version of Sherman sarcastically jests with Hampton, "Why most certainly, a man of your worth and character will be righteously considered when this war is finally over."

They all sit and begin discussing the final plan.

TRAIN STATION – TELEGRAPH OFFICE

Emo walks in to the telegraph office and finds the clerk casually relaxing with his feet propped up on a desk reading a newspaper. The clerk looks over the top of his paper and lowers his face to see what appears to be an Asian traveling salesman over the top of his spectacles.

"Can I help you?"

Emo pulls out a contraption out of his back pack. It's a small telegraph machine converted to a charger, among other things. He then pulls out his primitive two-way phone and a porcelain container with wires and tubes attached.

"I am Professor Emo. I have something you need. Instant breakfast machine. How you like your eggs?"

PLANTATION PROPERTY – CURRENT TIME

Datsuki is in the van monitoring the portal's energy in the equipment van by the creek, while also mixing his hip hop music. He is completely unaware of the time difference around him that his companions transported to, awaiting to hear on his two-way from Emo for further assistance. They both knew that Emo's receiver could not hold but a short charge and would require electricity to communicate.

Meanwhile, they had developed a solar flare simulator ready to go in case of emergency. It would send a strong pulse to generate enough frequency to both keep the portal and their bodies in sync. Hopefully, they would be back in time not to have to use it, as they hadn't tested it yet. Emo had calculated 20 hours max, but his figures weren't always exact. The burnt roast duck was just one example. There were hundreds of other failed experiments he neglected to tell Daniel or Brandy, and this was his grandest one of all.

"Pops, can you talk back yet? Hello?" Datsuki notices a small drop of energy levels on his monitor. He needed Emo to tell him at what level was critical enough to send the pulse. Meanwhile, he goes back to his twin turntables blasting music until he hears from pops.

DUNLAP HOME MEETING PLACE

Hampton confers with Sherman, "Our prisoners will be released this night as agreed at Ft. Donnelly."

"Agreed. And you sir, 2,000 within this night to be loaded onto the train, fed properly, and transported to our undisclosed location."

Hampton takes a swig. "Precisely. Oh, this is good Brandy."

Sherman puffing more smoke as the two play it out when Wirz disrupts the flow.

"I still think we should wait for General Winder."

Brandy's disdain for this contemptuous weasel is about to boil over. Hampton notices and is quick to reply. "Not necessary, why... he's liable to be on some wild goose chase."

Wirz gets a curious look on his face. "He did leave with a battalion rather abruptly... a sudden departure after an unusual wire he received."

Sherman grins at Hampton as they inhale cigars. "Chasing them damn Yankees, no doubt."

Laughter among the two, but Wirz is now looking suspicious. "General Winder has spoken of you General Hampton, but he never mentioned that your leg had healed from that wound. Could I see that scar?"

Hampton looks at Sherman with concern. There's a nervous, brief hush, then there's a knock on the door. Wirz is momentarily distracted. "Yes, we're in a meeting."

An elderly Mrs. Dunlap peeks through the door. "I'm sorry, I was just bringing some cookies. I can come at another..."

"By all means," Hampton quickly interjects, "Come in. Let us taste of those reputable sweets."

Sherman sighs a relief along with Hampton as she enters. Wirz quickly grabs one then steps outside as she passes by to offer to the others while both Brandy and Hampton stand before she sets the tray on the table.

Wirz approaches the guard outside. "You ride like the wind and find Winder. Tell him to get back here immediately." He gives him a few more words then sends him on his way. Shakespeare just quietly observes as Wirz goes back inside.

Mrs. Dunlap's hospitality is on display. "Is there anything else I can get you? Tea, sandwiches?"

Brandy wipes his mouth properly with a napkin, "These are delicious, my wife would appreciate the recipe."

"Oh, I would be delighted. You must miss her cooking."

Wirz is getting antsy. Mrs. Dunlap seems comfortable hosting a Union general and ready for more conversation. "Thank you, Mrs. Dunlap. You're most gracious, but..." Wirz hurries her.

"It's been nice meeting you both, please don't hesitate to call upon me for..."

Wirz begins to escort her out and cuts her off before she can complete her offer.

"We will. Thank you." She leaves and Wirz seems to have put his concern on hold. "Where were we?"

Brandy grabs a pen "Now, let us sign first, dispatch the orders and we have plenty of time to go over a few war stories with our good Captain here, right General."

"Indeed sir, proceed Captain, as the General here still has 60,000 troops at his command just hours from here."

Sherman looks at Wirz with a shit eating grin then sticks the cigar in his mouth. Wirz acquiesces and begins the process. "So I was told in your letter. If you'll both sign here and here, I will begin the exodus."

Sherman winks at Hampton as he takes another cookie from a stack and pushes it over to Hampton who indulges with a smile. They both grab a pen.

STOCKADE CONTINUOUS

The sun begins its descent toward the Eastern, sloping horizon beyond the stockade. Dark storm clouds roll in from the West. Inside the Montgomery tent, one man is trying to grasp the alternate world he's viewing while turning the pages of a *Life* Magazine from the 20th Century. James is going through a bevy of pictures of modern life, car advertisements, movie stars, black Americans, modern appliances, world events, then looks over at Daniel.

"This is proof enough. If you're not from the future, maybe you're an angel."

"I'm your great, great grandson."

James is bewildered, at the same time, overwhelmed, as he embraces Daniel with a strong hug.

"There's more…" He breaks out a copy of a 100-year Anniversary of the Civil War Edition *National Geographic*. "James, God as my witness, you and your brave soldiers saved this country from ruin and ended slavery for good. You died to set men free and preserve the Union."

James turns the pages as Daniel goes on. "Your suffering and the harsh cruelties of war were never more documented and preserved as in this war between the states. Our United States of America honors your bravery and tradition with battle reenactments and memorial services, year after year - both North and South. Life around the entire world is a better place because of what happened here over the course of four agonizing years. More than one million wounded and almost 800,000 dead paved the way, more than all the future wars to come combined."

James is wiping his tears.

"We try to wrap our heads around what you and your families are all going through. But I swear, nothing in our history has ever, nor will ever, compare to this deplorable mass of inhumane abyss as Andersonville. Do you have any idea how many men are in here now?"

'No sir."

"More than 30,000, they just carried out more than 100 dead today. We've got to get you out of here."

James gets up and ponders.

Now that Daniel has convinced him of the future, he begins to inquire about the past. "Why are you pictured as a sergeant when it's become clear that you are a high-ranking officer?"

He looks out his tent. Daniel is even more curious about his other mysterious ancestor. "And your letters, no return address to your wife Rachel. Does she still live in Missouri?"

James continues to look out, then casually answers, "No, she lives near the capital to be near her father and work in the hospital."

"Her father?"

Suddenly, James turns with the most perplexed look on his face. Daniel is acutely aware of this sudden change in demeanor. "Yes, her father, the President."

Daniel's jaw drops.

James A. Montgomery, completely surprised, exclaims, "You don't know?! My God man, her father is Abraham Lincoln!"

Daniel stands up and drops everything to the ground. He stares in disbelief around the tent.

James, now deeply troubled, asks, "How can this be? Yes, he has delayed her identity up to now, but has sworn to her he will reveal her true identity because the child she's carrying demands it - just as soon as the election is over. He's a good man. If you're from the future you would know this. Unless…" Daniel's thoughts are racing. "…something happens. Daniel, tell me please, what could it be?"

Daniel is now fitting the pieces of the puzzle. "*You're* the VIP! That's why they're looking for you. The President, and all the President's men. They just don't know exactly why."

"I had to disguise myself and my rank, up until now. Her life was in danger from being kidnapped at the beginning of his presidency and the South eager to overturn his election. A small Confederate conspiracy was rumored as someone in their ranks has known her since childhood in Louisiana. The blackmail, smear, or even the threat of murder, could've compromised the stability of the Union. They even captured me once, held me prisoner waiting for terms of ransom, but I escaped… not before I relieved them of their treasonous lives."

"You killed them?"

James just looks blankly with the answer unspoken. Daniel begins to sit back down and pats the bed.

"Louisiana? Sit. You must tell me all about it."

TELEGRAPH OFFICE

Emo has convinced the clerk to let him give a demonstration, as he has wired his remodeled telegraph machine to the electrical wiring. Emo understands at that day and time the electrical current was only a one-way system, that is how the signals were sent. He's prepared his to convert it so it will charge his two-way in order to communicate to number one son back at the van.

Suddenly, Datsuki's voice comes over the air waves. "Pops, you hooked up yet?"

The clerk nearly falls out of his seat at the sound if his voice. Emo grabs the wired phone box.

"I'm a genius! You coming in loud and clear." Emo turns to the clerk. "Now I show you how it cooks."

"I need help with these readings," Datsuki replies over the two-way as music blares in the background.

The clerk is spellbound. "To hell with that, I know how to cook. How in the tarnation is that thing talking to you?"

Emo smiles, now he knows it's charging and he has connection.

STOCKADE

Inside the tent, James tells what he knows of the background of Daniel's newly discovered ancestor. "Louisiana, yes, during Lincoln's youth, he met her mother on his river journeys to New Orleans. She was among what they called the "antebellum status" of the colored community. They pride themselves on their education, their breeding, and wealth. They had a brief affair before he departed and promised to see her again, but it was not to be. He fell in love with another up North and never returned. He found out years later as Rachel's mother paid him a secret visit. He was obliged at the time to honor her as his child, but not wanting to destroy his reputation, her mother kept in communication and agreed later would be a proper time."

"I'm listening," and he was intently so as not to miss a single detail. "So, tell me about Rachel. She sounds most enchanting."

"Ah, Rachel. She is my love, my life." James pulls out a portrait of a beautiful, olive skinned, dark- haired young woman of sophistication "She was educated in Europe and has such a gift for writing. Her father, who loves poetry himself, introduced her to Walt Whitman who tutored and encouraged her."

"This is all coming together," Daniel figures. James then hands the tintype to Daniel. Almost immediately he recognizes the dress pattern and matching bonnet in her lap, then stares into the face he so longed to see in that unforgettable meadow. "Lavender girl! I've seen her, gathering flowers..."

"How is that possible?" James asks perplexed.

"She's the reason I'm here...with you. I needed a sign if to go on, with this portal...just when things seemed impossible, I turned another corner, another page."

"You mentioned lavender. She gathers the delicate flowers and dries the petals... that's her favorite." James smells the fragrance from her letter and hands it to Daniel.

"Yes, I'm familiar with that now. A sweet smell now embedded with a vision of her."

James chuckles. "You're like her, putting everything you experience into fancy words." He hesitates and recalls, "Except for her voice, her accent, that's what captured me at first."

"How so?" Daniel inquires further, wanting more details.

'Well, imagine a Cajun educated in England. She also claimed to have met her grandfather in France."

Daniel now notices James slight Midwest drawl. "Tell me of that first time meeting her."

"We met after I was graduated from West Point near the capital. She caught my eye at a ball. I lost contact, when suddenly she came up behind me, tapped me on my shoulder and began the most poetic advances on a man I have ever seen, in that charming accent. Needless to say, I was swooned by her. We immediately fell in love and shortly after, became engaged. The night I proposed, I insisted on asking her father first. I had no idea what I was asking." James gets up and starts smiling, then becomes animated as he tells this story. "She starts laughing."

Daniel is getting a visual.

"Can you imagine? I was insisting on asking the hand of the secret daughter of President Abraham Lincoln."

Daniel is chuckling.

"This wonderful creature started toying with me. "Are you a Republican?" she'd ask. "He prefers speeches. Can you prepare a state of the union while asking for my hand?"

Daniel is laughing. "She is something. Your head must have been spinning by now."

"Yes! All I wanted to do was the gentlemanly thing, and she's making fun of me. So, we take a carriage across town to the White House area and she says, "Here we are." "Well," I said, "here we are where?" And, she says, "My father's house."

He makes a face of Okay... "Oh, I understand. Well, it's okay if your father is a servant, I still love you and someday we'll have servants of our own, I promised. After she regains her composure from laughing, she breaks down and tells me her father is Abraham Lincoln. By now, I don't know what to believe. Maybe I'm marrying a crazy woman."

James rubs his cheek then remembers. "There was a lot of security at that time. His life was threatened daily.

She hands a guard a note, then we walk to view the garden from a safe distance. Shortly, out walks Mr. Lincoln into the garden. It's getting dark and the guard escorts us over to him and I notice he expresses a warm gesture to her, but not affectionate. She looks at me after introducing me. Daniel…I forgot why I was there. She looks at me, then him. He then starts smiling. "You're a graduate of high rank at West Point?" he inquires. She then takes my hand and he understands. He walks me alone for a few minutes and expresses his deep, but conflicted affections for her. I am moved that he confides in me his care for her future. I swore allegiance to this family secret and we walk back. She sees the smile on his face and can no longer keep reserve, so she hugs and kisses him. We were married shortly after, then this war called me away."

"Were you captured once before and escaped?" Daniel needed to know.

"Just the kidnapping I mentioned, not imprisoned. One escaped the blade of my knife. Booth was his name, a devious traitor who was always hatching plots."

Daniel's alarm bells are swirling but he dare not mention his recognition of the assassin. He'd delve into that with him later. Daniel was somewhat aware but now confirmed what history had discovered. Booth's original plan was to kidnap Lincoln, but they just didn't know how far back and deep it went.

"That's too bad, if only you had succeeded…" There's an awkward moment of silence, then Daniel presses on with his questioning.

"Did you impregnate her upon a leave?" Daniel was pressing deeper to verify the family suspicion.

James, a bit startled, "How did you know that? It's true. One blissful night in D. C., then I was hurried back. Are you married Daniel? Children?"

"My wife's name is Michelle. We have no children."

James seems a bit disturbed. "Please Daniel, tell me."

Daniel is alert.

"Will I see my child?"

Daniel hesitates. Suddenly, there's a big stir outside that takes both their attention and they both step out.

There's a lot of movement stirring when a private runs up to James.

"What's going on Casey?" asks Montgomery.

"They're rounding up 2,000 men to be transferred. We got one hour. Only the healthy and fittest."

Daniel remarks, "That would be my colleagues, we're getting you and 2,000 men out of here by train."

"Where are they taking us?"

"To freedom."

THE PLANTATION

Inside Daniel's manor things begin transforming back to its original state. Victorian art and furniture slowly begin morphing into the contemporary furniture Daniel had placed. The portal moves along a horizontal plane and it's obviously beginning to disappear as it approaches the kitchen and the upstairs master bedroom. Oblivious to the interior, Datsuki is outside alarmed by the readings showing even a greater drop in frequency. He stops his turntables and grabs the two- way.

"Pops, you are losing energy! What do I do? You ok?"

TELERAPH OFFICE

As the clerk is amazed watching eggs and bacon cooking in a porcelain container, he now observes coffee beginning to drip into a cup. Emo grabs the transmitter box upon hearing Datsuki.

"Sorry, gotta go."

"What about your contraption?"

"You keep. No charge."

Emo flees the office outside to a train pulling in the station.

"That's one crazy Chinaman."

The clerk smells the bacon, but doesn't realize, Emo has disabled all wiring and communication that will take them days to reconfigure. The Confederates are cut off.

TRAIN STATION - CONTINUOUS

Dark clouds are forming a storm as Union soldiers are boarding the train in droves. Rebel soldiers are waving lanterns and calling out to board while Brandy and Emo are by a train car entry no longer in disguise. Forrester is on the train looking out the window. Abruptly, there's another energy surge, this time twice as flashing and more pronounced. Brandy and Emo look at each other.

"Time for emergency generator. You find Daniel. We got to hurry now."

Brandy starts heading toward the prison against the crowd, looking at everyone. He makes his way until closer to the wall when he spots Shakespeare still in his rebel Private uniform. "Where's Daniel?" Brandy asks.

"I don't know, he was at the gate with his relative then I lost him. I'm boarding."

Thunder RUMBLES. He leaves and Brandy stares at the gate. One side is closing. "God no."

THE PLANTATION

Emo's son is furiously adjusting equipment. "Son... hello? (static) "Datsuki, you need to blast solar flare now!" Emo pleas over the speaker.

The solar flare simulator is generating off the engine from the van with a satellite dish aiming at a slightly upward angle. Datsuki runs and checks everything as he hears Emo calling.

"Hurry! We need blast now!"

Datsuki grabs the two- way "OK, OK! I'll blast now."

He pulls the lever and a sonic BOOM fills the air. The trees bend and animals flee.

"We did it! Readings are back up."

Datsuki looks over and sees smoke billowing from the simulator. It's melting. Meanwhile inside the manor, the portal has moved beyond the interior and has traveled almost to the creek but has stopped. The outside of the mansion is morphing back into the house and deck Daniel originally stood on that unforgettable morning.

ANDERSONVILLE OUTSKIRTS COUNTRYSIDE

A troop of Cavalry is trotting quickly with General Winder who is leading the pack cursing to the officer next to him. "When I get my hands on the idiot who sent me on a wild goose chase after some Yankee ghosts, I'll have his head."

"Yes sir."

A rider from Andersonville, the guard, visible in the distant skyline, quickly approaches. General Winder raises his hand to stop all behind him as the rider pulls up, physically winded.

"General Winder, Sir." catching his breath.

"Well, what is it soldier?"

His horse is restless. "Captain Wirz...he says General Hampton is here. He signed a prisoner exchange."

"Hampton! He's 200 miles from here in the Carolinas. What prisoner exchange?"

"Hundreds sir, boarding the train now."

Winder looks at the skyline and sees locomotive smoke rising. He's furious. It starts to rain.

STOCKADE CAMP

At the gate in the spurting rain, Daniel is beseeching James to come with him, as the last of the soldiers are leaving.

Daniel is pleading with James "This is your last chance; the train is leaving."

"I can't leave my men, they'll die if I don't get them out soon."

Daniel is looking at James, then at the gate. They're ready to close. There's chaos everywhere as men now start flooding toward the gate. SHOTS are fired in the air.

Brandy is yelling from outside, "Daniel! Come on!"

Daniel turns to see Brandy amongst the crowd outside then back at James. Daniel pleas with him.

"You go! I have another plan. You just leave. I have to do this," James insists.

Daniel starts toward the gate when he watches James turn and head back to his area. The gate is closing. Daniel sees Brandy with a look of lost hope as the gate finally closes with Daniel inside. THUNDER ROARS. The rain is pouring.

TRAIN STATION

Emo is urgently assisting passengers to board with his freshly charged radio. "Get on. Quickly!"

The walkie talkie blares his son's voice. "Pops, readings are up but going down again slowly... maybe abort soon. Machine blowup!"

Emo notices Captain Wiz coming through with a couple of men so he rushes to the engineer.

"We go now! No more time. Go!"

The engineer hustles and yells orders to his conductor to get on. Emo starts looking for his companions. Shakespeare is approaching the train to board, wearing full dress with a gray cape, when he is stopped by Wirz. "Where's General Hampton?"

"Not sure, sir."

"Where are you going? You stand here until I find Hampton."

He looks at the two with Wirz and obeys. Wirz moves down the line as the train starts moving.

General Winder is trotting into town with troops and sees the train a short distance starting to whistle and leave. "This way! Stop that train!"

The band of about twenty hard riding rebel Cavalry head on a gallop to stop the train.

At the train station, Brandy finds Emo on a car opening and walks beside him as it moves. "Daniel didn't make it. We got to go to plan B." Emo is staring in disbelief. Brandy realizes the danger when they both look back and see a charging Cavalry. He orders Emo, "It's too dangerous, you might miss the portal. I'll handle it. You go on."

Datsuki's voice comes over the two- way, "No time showing. You in red zone! Maybe only hour...maybe..." just then, it cuts out.

Emo is distracted while analyzing the situation when Brandy stops walking as the train slowly pulls away, waving goodbye to Emo. The rain stops. "I got this," Brandy says to himself. Emo watches as Brandy turns and heads away.

Winder and his troops race forward and continue closing in. Shakespeare sees his chance as Wirz and the two guards are distracted. He runs and jumps onto the car then smugly salutes a frustrated Wirz watching him pass. "I'll have you hanged!"

General Winder gasps, ordering fervently, "Stop the train!" His Cavalry charges up to the train and follow from the side of the rear car. Winder stays behind and rides up to Wirz. "What the devil's going on here?" yells a livid Winder.

"It appears to be a grand escape sir."

The Cavalry have caught up with most of the train. They maneuver to start boarding, then a few SHOTS are fired. Shakespeare realizes if they board, they will start gunning down men until they reach the engineer and stop the train. He steps to the edge of an open car and jumps on the rebel's horse, throwing him off under the train wheels. He flips around facing backward while riding, unfurls his cape, whips out two Colt revolvers then rapidly unloads twelve rounds, ripping into the unsuspecting pursuing Cavalry. They quickly begin falling over dead, left and right, until the few that remain riding disband and retreat. Shakespeare jumps back on the train. Winder looks on as he loses the train, as well as half his men. It's gone. Brandy smiles as he hears the angry exchange between Wirz and Winder, then turns to leave the station area. Barrister had failed to mention Shakespeare was a gunslinger also.

Brandy mumbles to himself, "Grand escape indeed. This calls for a toast." He lights a cigar and strolls down main street Andersonville. He approaches a local resident. "Say, you got a bar around here?"

"There's a saloon in the feed and tackle store."

Brandy eyes the feed store and humors himself, "Great. So, my horse can enjoy happy hour with me."

STOCKADE CAMP - NIGHT

The Georgia rain begins again. Inside, many of the men who are dying of thirst open their mouths, or hold out containers to catch the water drops. Daniel is with James at a makeshift infirmary area that begins to flood. The downpours have always been a blessing, as well as a curse. They pull one immobilized soldier out of drowning pool swirling around his head, as others organized an evacuation to another area on safer ground, which is already overcrowded. James explains to Daniel, as they move the helpless bodies, "We had an escape plan of our own. We have to evacuate about 25 sick men from my company. I couldn't leave them. They'll be dead in a week."

"I understand, I've interfered again," he said softly, remembering the blood bath on Sugar Hill.

"They will be on the alert now. We'll have to move out tonight. There are three wagons waiting about two miles outside down at the East basin."

"What can I do?"

A soldier runs up to Montgomery, "They're ready Major. Two are on the outside already."

"You can help get these men to the south wall," he insists to Daniel. "Come, I'll show you."

They head toward an area near a wall where they've been digging and securing an escape tunnel for weeks. It seems well-planned, with each man having a specific duty. Daniel realizes his ancestor has a natural leadership quality with a profound respect by his men under his command. From what Brandy had explained to him, there were a few small groups who held together, but for the most part, inside this primitive den, it was every man for himself.

Daniel lifts a man who is unbelievably weak and fragile while another soldier comes along to help. The rain is pouring down fiercely, moving mud and streams of sludge everywhere while lots of activity begins swirling around the escape area. They bring the weakened soldier to a team, bundling them up in blankets and rope, just before getting pulled through a tunnel where the line is attached to a group on the outside. James points for Daniel to help another soldier wrapped in a blanket while another quickly knots the rope.

"That's good. I've got it from here." The soldier tugs hard and Daniel watches as the wrapped soldier disappears.

Two more bundled men barely make it out, just before there's a flurry of commotion.

A Sergeant runs up with grave alarm shouting, "Pull the cover. I think they're coming."

They stop their action and pull a tent over the hole. Several helpless men are left waiting to get through as James runs up carrying his saber. Daniel is staring at it, remembering their conversation how he managed to conceal it.

MONTGOMERY TENT – EARLIER

"Now you understand? Had they known my identity, eventually it would have complicated matters and possibly compromised the President's decisions. They would've put me in a separate enlisted men's camp not far from here."

"Yet you would've fared much better there than this death camp; that was valiant of you."

"At one time, I was offered a safe command near the Potomac, but I would have none of that." James went on to give Daniel a history of his father and upbringing. His military exploits and his heritage were expressed with great pride. Also, a fondness for his mother and siblings was obvious. He was very much a family man who was looking forward to being a father and raising a family were his life circumstance different than it was. This opened Daniel's eyes to a newfound perspective of his bloodline. James continued, "In the field behind the lines, I was a Major in command. Upon my last assigned mission, I changed into my role as Sergeant and left my belongings behind not far from here. Only my commanding General was advised, yet he didn't know fully why."

"That explains your sword, of higher rank. Speaking of, how would I've come into possession of it? It was handed down to me since my mother died."

James looks a little perplexed and a bit disconcerted. "That gives me the strangest feeling, Daniel. My death... possessions..." He stands and walks over to the opening of his tent. "Perhaps my being here...instead of remaining near Rachel, was a mistake."

How uncanny, Daniel thought the same about Michelle. Now he was searching for an answer, but could only wonder the outcome if his escape plan would work, to save his ancestor and alter the chain of events for the next century. James then reaches under his cot to pull out the saber that Daniel immediately recognized as the one handed down to him.

"This must be to what you're referring," James says very calmly.

He immediately recognizes it. "There are no blood stains on it."

James continues, "My men who remained on the outside saw to it that it, among a few letters between Rachel and I, made it through the tunnel. They urged me to escape. But as you can see, I'm needed here. We kept thinking, surely a prisoner exchange was coming soon. However, your silence regarding the question of my future since your arrival has awakened me to a lesser fate."

STOCKADE – SOUTH WALL TUNNEL PRESENT

The Sergeant under Montgomery runs up to the escape operation and surrounding area and yells wildly, "Battle formation! They're coming! Everyone take position!"

Several men pull out makeshift weapons and knives then head toward the enemy.

"Daniel, wait in my tent."

"No way. Give me a weapon." he demands without hesitation.

James looks at Daniel and smiles proudly. "A writer turned soldier. Let's fight together!" He looks back over his shoulder and yells to those remaining and waiting to be tunneled out, "Open it up and get them all through now!"

A SHOT rings out. James sees the tower guard aiming outside at the escapees and races toward the foot of the tower. Another SHOT fires at a distance from the outside and a tower guard falls to his death on the ground. A troop of rebel guards comes running toward the south wall with bayonets facing out.

The Sergeant can be heard yelling, "Come 'ere, you bastards. Charge!"

Suddenly, the rebels are outnumbered by all the men rising up and coming out of nowhere. Toward the other wall, James, Daniel, and the armed men are charging another group of rebel guards when he's knocked dizzy to the ground. Another SHOT is fired and a union soldier is dropped in the deadline. Daniel shakes it off, gets up, then sees James climbing the tower as a rebel drops dead next to him from a knife wound. Daniel grabs his rifle. The tower guard sees James climbing and aims his rifle. Daniel yells at the guard, firing the weapon, but he misses. That distracts long enough for James to climb in the tower and engage in a hand-to-hand combat. The sword finally drives through the rebel's body and he falls out of the tower. James salutes Daniel then waves his saber for the men to keep escaping, as he can see the getaway wagons below on the outside. He then begins to climb down. "Carry on. Keep going."

Daniel is watching him with reverence, when suddenly just feet from him, a SHOT fires and strikes James. Daniel, with two other men, converge on the rebel and he is immediately stabbed and bayoneted from three sides; he drops dead and left bloodied. Now James is wounded, becomes weaker, and falls the rest of the way. They quickly rush to his aid to find him barely conscious.

Daniel pleas with others, "Do you men have any kind of doctor in here?"

"No. I'm okay, just get me to my bed."

"Get him to his tent then," Daniel commands.

In the aftermath, the rain has almost ceased outside while Daniel is seated on the bed of his dying ancestor who lies near a flickering candle.

James softly encourages him, "We got 'em out didn't we?"

"We sure did, they will live to see their families. I'll help get you..."

"Daniel, I know my fate. I saw it in your eyes." He takes his Bible from his bed stand.

Daniel listens closely to James' spiritual side "Christ died to set men free. We die fighting for the right to believe it."

Daniel is moved, now he can only hopelessly wait.

"In my book, there's a map. Please, could you get it?"

Daniel reaches for his book and finds a map.

"Before I was captured, I hid my troop movements and battle orders in a leather satchel in an old oak tree hollow near our last night's encampment." He points to an area. "There you'll find her diary, some poetry, and a letter from Lincoln written to her, confirming he's her father."

"A letter? Why did you have all her...?"

"She wanted me to have them. She was afraid no one would ever believe her story. Daniel, write her story."

Daniel slips the map inside his shirt as he watches his eyes close. James A. Montgomery breathes his last breath. Daniel takes a moment thoughtfully, then he puts the blanket over his head and snuffs out the candle.

Bring Out Your Dead

ANDERSONVILLE STOCKADE PRISON GATE

The rain and clouds have cleared and a bright moon lights the night. They are bringing out the dead and piling onto a wagon. The guard waves them on as they pull away to the Hades of Andersonville cemetery for their final place of rest.

ANDERSONVILLE - TAVERN

Brandy is passed out on a table by a half empty bottle from drinking. A saloon keeper wakes him. "You, wake up."

Brandy lifts his head and realizes he's late. "What time is it?"

"After midnight."

He sees an old clock standing behind the bar that reads 12:15. "Daniel!" He jumps up and runs out looking both ways to regain his bearings. He walks up to the prison gate and realizes there are no bodies. Only one guard remains, smoking a stump of a cigar. "Where's the burying detail?"

"Burying the dead, where else?"

Brandy grabs a shovel and runs.

CEMETERY - MOMENTS LATER

Brandy finds the row they're currently using. The grave detail are done and just leaving. There's about twenty markers. Brandy begins furiously digging when suddenly a gun pokes his head from behind.

"Whattya think you're doin'?" a ragged scavenger interrupts. Brandy slowly turns. There are two grave robbers disguised as guards with rifles aiming directly toward him.

"We's kill grave robbers." says the other.

"My friend, he's not dead?" implores Brandy.

"We shoot crazy people, too." They both break out laughing.

"I'm not crazy, I'm a Harvard professor."

"And I'm Napoleon Bonaparte. You can just start diggin' your own grave."

Brandy, under the point of their guns, begins to dig, when out of nowhere the familiar accent of Professor Emo is heard demanding, "Now drop guns down, Johnny reb. You die."

Emo cocks the pistol. Click. Brandy sees Emo and is relieved. "You didn't leave!"

"Been trying to find you pin head. Where you been?"

"Looking for Chinese take-out. No time now, we gotta find Daniel?"

Emo pulls out his squawking meter startling the rebels, thinking it's a futuristic weapon, they drop their rifles and take off running like yellow-bellied cowards. Emo immediately begins running over the graves with his meter. "How many you say?"

"20… maybe 50."

"You guess like Vegas."

Emo's meter reads loud and clear after about ten covered graves. They both begin to dig furiously - Brandy with a shovel, and Emo, with his hands flinging dirt in the air from the other end. Within seconds, Emo finds a passed-out Daniel, barely breathing. They uncover him and he gasps for fresh air and becomes conscious. He sits up after a few moments then realizes the plan has worked. He's alive and out of the prison.

"I'm so sorry Daniel, I screwed up. I should've ..." Brandy searches for the right words.

"He's alive!" Exclaims Emo.

"Yes, that I am." He stares back at the line of graves, then toward the stockade of Andersonville Prison. "I will never forget this valley of walking bones as long as I live."

After a moment of reflecting on Daniel's vivid summary, Brandy counters with their victory, "Well, if it's of any consequence, we did save 2,000 lives."

Daniel alters his dire reflection to one of enthusiasm. He pulls out his ancestor's saber from his pant leg. "So it worked! We altered history!"

"I never saw such joy for life as on that train," Brandy affirms with pride.

Daniel puts his arms around the two of them, and as they walk off together he begins to lightly sing, "This train...carries broken-hearted. This train, carries souls departed, oh this train, will not be thwarted, for this train, faith will be rewarded. Yes, this train, hear the big wheels singing...This train bells of freedom ringing."

Emo inquires, "Shakespeare?"

"Springsteen," Daniel replies flatly.

The air is fresh and clear. A bright morning sun warms the slight mist coming up from the moist ground. A train is pulling in, puffing steam and cranking to a slow halt in the much emptier station, contrasting from the day before.

Under a large tree, the three time travelers are observing the train from a distant grove. Daniel is holding a horse by the reins, along with Rachel's trinket around his wrist.

Emo gives an update, "Son say no more generator. My theory last day for portal. We lucky, sun flare up, give more time."

Brandy jokes, "Fortune cookie say, he who fly naked upside down have hairy crack up...."

Daniel laughs with Brandy.

"Time warp your brain like bad chop suey - all noodle no meat."

Brandy makes a fist.

"That's gonna be a long train ride back for you two. Brandy, take care of his saber for me. Gentlemen, according to the map, I've got a two-hour ride, then an hour home." Daniel hops on his horse.

Brandy pulls out a flask. "See you in 2015." Brandy toasts, "Here's to a hundred and fifty years, and the bloodline of Abraham Lincoln!"

"You drink too much, like fish." Emo acknowledges.

Brandy swigs, then wipes his pants with it. "Fish this you slant-eyed nerd."

Daniel rides off as they continue bantering, walking toward the train station.

After riding over an hour, he comes to a hill and stops to look at the map again. Wondering if he's drifted too far, he looks up and sees a large oak tree from a distance and takes off trotting. A reverse surge of energy flashes stronger than ever, as he begins prompting the horse to go faster. Just as he approaches a SHOT ricochet's off the tree then another SHOT spooks the horse and flips Daniel to the ground. He sees four raiders approaching from a hill, then he looks at the tree and sees the hollow opening where James mentioned. He starts on foot for the tree when a round of SHOTS are fired again, preventing Daniel from reaching the tree just by a few feet. If he crawls and tries to hide behind the large oak trunk, they'll trap him for sure.

He's forced to save his life and goes for his horse, then hops on and gallops as swiftly as he can. It's too dangerous to wait and hide as the portal reverse surges again, so he flees in the opposite direction and heads for home.

MANOR CURRENT TIME

Emo and his son are trying to repair equipment and busy monitoring data. The portal has left his manor and retreated back across the creek. Upon hearing the horse with Daniel racing over the hill, Emo yells for him to hurry. Daniel sees his house is in 2015 and realizes the time portal divide is obviously back to the creek line. The reverse surge is almost stationary. He can see Emo jumping and yelling, "Hurry Daniel!" Emo frantically urges him. He turns to his son, "More energy!" Datsuki is in the van running a hand crank as fast as possible as Daniel is cutting through the forest when he watches the bridge disappear. The horse rears up as Daniel makes one last run to leap over the creek. "Keep going, he almost here!"

The portal reverses for good just behind Daniel, as his horse leaps across the creek and disappears underneath him. Daniel flies through the air and rolls to the foot of Emo. He stands up and brushes himself off in disbelief.

"You lucky... You in time for dinna!"

They look at each other, then at the charred duck on a platter, by the van. They all start laughing.

Daniel then notices and thinks to ask, "Where's Brandy?"

Emo looks back over the creek as Daniel also looks out. "He stayed. No come back."

That familiar breeze picks up and the last of the fall leaves twirl to the ground. The time portal is gone.

Daniel Summary

T he following day, in a modern suburb, a giant, leafless oak tree stands out in a small green belt among dozens of recently built homes. Its web of branches, limbs and twigs gives it such character it demands a name. Daniel drives around a winding road up to the entry way where he spots the same tree he tried to reach 150 years ago, or was it just yesterday. Nevertheless, he's relieved to discover that at least there still might be a chance the treasure he was seeking is still in that giant oak, now twice as large, and higher than before. He pulls up and gets out of his car to look up the tree but can't tell if the hollow remained all this time. He sees a utility worker down the block on a bucket lift. *What are the chances?* he figures.

After buying the workers lunch, one is in the bucket reaching into a hole and pulls out the crusty, but preserved leather satchel. He looks down with a big smile from his find and sees Daniel dancing with delight. The tree was given a name, and has been known ever since as The Dancing Tree.

Pacing on the deck, Daniel is on the landline phone with his agent while he's looking at her diary, letters, and poems laid out on a table, along with the watch he found by the creek which belonged to Sarah. Separated among them is a hand-written letter penned by Abraham Lincoln, certifying that Rachel Emma Montgomery, was indeed his daughter.

"Jason, I've got my story."

"I never doubted you for a minute."

An incoming call interrupts the call with an incessant click.

"Hold on, I got another call... Hello?"

Michelle is on the line. "Daniel. God, it's good to hear your voice."

"Michelle, your voice sounds wonderful, too."

In their Los Angles bedroom, under a bright light, she rolls over on the bed and sits up. She's glowing from ear to ear. "Daniel, please be happy when I tell you this."

He continues pacing, "I'm all ears."

"I'm pregnant!"

Daniel raises the phone sky high and yells with glee as he slips into a happy dance.

"Daniel...is that good?" Michelle asks meekly.

"I'm the happiest man in the world. I could kiss you a thousand times."

Jason interjects, "That's wonderful Daniel, but you couldn't pay me enough."

Michelle laughs, "Come home, Daniel. We all miss you."

Daniel puts down the phone, picks up the diary, and holds it to his chest along with Rachel's trinket then walks to the deck railing for a final farewell. It's completely silent. Just then a noise from above draws his attention. He looks up and sees a flock of geese flying over in prefect formation.

GRAVEYARD FROM OPENING SCENE –
ONE YEAR LATER

Leaves continue falling to the ground and blow by the grave of the ancestor, Rachel Emma Montgomery, next to a newly erected monument, Rachel Lincoln Montgomery. Daniel is standing by his wife and baby on a platform as he opens a page from his book, in front of a seated crowd and gathered media. He reads a poem from her most painful period, after the death and funeral of Abraham Lincoln. It was discovered among Whitman's archives.

As spoken in Rachel's voice:

When I sleep, there are places I remember
With fondness close to tender
It brings to bear with affection
In my life those persons I recollect
But none more than you my beloved
Does the impression deepen to such an effect

Is not the heart meant for holding the finest gain?
With each breath, I anticipate
The final release of this lingering pain
To lastly be only occupied with love

Oh, this dying day
A funeral passes my way
Dark and dreary a nation mourns
They've lost their martyr of the free
But I have lost a father
A husband, and a future without glee

Daniel's voice:

But when I awoke I was not alone
For there was a child next to me
To carry on the God within thee.

And that's how it was in the fall of 1864, and in the fall of my life. My novel, *Diary of an Ancestor*, categorized as historical fiction, is a controversial best seller. Even though DNA had proven my story, there will always be skeptics. Can you blame them? As it turns out, Rachel <u>was</u> in Washington D.C., working tirelessly in the many hospitals and medical camps that had come to fill the city during the Civil War. This is where she grew her friendship with Walt Whitman, as he was committed to helping the soldiers in this capacity also. It's understandable how one could either be repulsed by the horrors of war upon these men never to revisit, or be completely engrossed with compassion, as was the daughter of Abraham Lincoln, her dearest father, and Walt Whitman, her father and tutor of her passion - writing. She could be near both, and caring for each soldier, as if vicariously it could be her beloved husband, James A. Montgomery. These medical facilities varied in size, profession, and cleanliness. But none can deny, aside from her dedication and service, Americans came together to care for their sons, as there were soldiers from both sides in that not so civilized war, and both sides equally deserved care and dignity.

Besides the letters and poems I discovered which James had hidden, obviously before his death, I also acquired her writings and a latter diary that was mixed in with the estate and collections of Walt Whitman. No one knew who she was. Whitman knew, but he took it to his grave. He was loyal to the President and knowledge of her after his death would've only tarnished a nation's respect for the finest President who had presided over the most difficult time in our history.

Sadly, Rachel died three years after the war ended, most probably of a broken heart, never knowing of his heroic last stand or his final breaths. Her son, my great grandfather, was raised by the Whitman family, whom I never knew, but thanks to the time portal, I now know my heritage, ancestry and my purpose. Is it any wonder then that I became a writer…and a happy father?

I am more than pleased and fulfilled to give her the voice she so passionately wanted the world to hear; to know of her life, her husband, of Whitman, and understandably, her true father. Here is an excerpt from her diary:

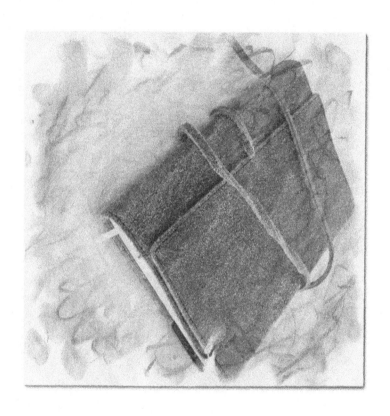

Diary of an Ancestor

F eb 12, 1864- This day at Armory-square, I finished
writing more letters than ever for these poor dear lads.
Though short, as I'm between tending the horribly wounded,
who's concern is first to stay alive rather than concern for
loved ones at home, yet long enough to convey their aching
of missing them so and of their sadness for the miles they
have apart. Some, even after recovery, linger in a state of
gray, so forlorn. They've given this state of illness a name
as of recent, homesick*, or homesickness. But the hardest
still are much beyond homesickness and closer to dying,
much more than are living. Besieged with such body count
since Fredericksburg, then Bull Run, I've since lost track
of names. Today, I have the blood drenched in my clothing
of at least twenty men. Hardly men, on average, 19, maybe
younger –or older, but much too premature to apprehend
such onslaught of heaviness upon their poor young souls
and ravaged bodies to face the face of death.

One such soldier from New York Infantry (his regiment
he told me, but I have since disregard for such detail), was
blown apart by artillery - can't even hear, his legs mangled
and prepared to be removed, could not let go of my hand. I
simply had to break free, as I am not allowed during ampu-
tations, I have since learned he pulled through, but may not

survive the night. I shall see him before I leave close to midnight, my usual time to rest and be safe in bed.

The word was coined during the Civil War to describe the deep 'nostalgia" for home and family. It was described as a mental health condition that soldiers actually died from.

Feb 13, 1864 - I began my morning by preparing biscuits and collecting pies my gracious ladies provide me, some even accompany me on my rounds. At the beginning, there were many medical camps, too numerous, so I've settled at the Armory-square - they are just as hungry there. The Northerners call me Madame Montgomery, the Southerners, Miss Rachel. They both are so lonely, kind, most quiet, but a few cannot stop talking once they know me. Many men survey the wounded. My dearest is Mr. Whitman, or "Uncle Walt" who attends daily, and well into the night, yet obvious some soldiers prefer the company of a woman, yet any at all is most appreciated. There are no complaints. They face death and pain the same, with brave certainty.

He shared with me of a letter he wrote to two fellow New Yorkers:

"Got very much interested in some cases in hospitals here - go now steadily to more or less of said hospitals by day or night- find always the sick and dying soldiers forthwith begin to cling to me in a way that makes a fellow feel funny enough. These hospitals, so different from all others- these thousands, and tens of twenty thousands of American young men, badly wounded, all sorts of wounds, operated on, pallid with diarrhea, languishing, dying with fever, pneumonia. open a new world to me, somehow, giving closer insights, new things. Exploring deeper mines, than any yet, showing our humanity tried

by terrible, fear fullest tests. Probed deepest, the living souls, the body's tragedies, bursting the petty bonds of art."

I shared a piece of pie with Uncle Walt this day at noon, he shared his newest poem, and I, mine with him. He helped me with the last two lines, words arranged so cleverly, he surpasses my skills, yet inspires me nonetheless. He too expresses, with utter disdain, the conditions in some medical camps: dreary, uncleanness to almost filth, short of attention, lacking food; he tends to sway authority when he comes across such neglect, I on the other hand take it upon myself to make a list and present it to father at the end of the week. I'm not sure whom he chooses to convey my recommendations, but most are carried out without further haste. Uncle Walt knows of my situation and is rather fond, if not fascinated, by my father's daily activities among the streets and affairs of Washington – yet, more profoundly, acutely aware of his humble and deep concern when he visits, which is quite often.

The gray bearded poet is very descriptive of my father's facial expressions, his appearance – *"I think well of the President. He has a face like a Hoosier Michel Angelo, so awful ugly it becomes beautiful, with its strange mouth, its deep cut, crisscross lines, and its doughnut complexion. My notion is, too, that underneath his outside mannerism, and stories from third class county barrooms (it is his humor), he has a tender side. Mr. Lincoln keeps a fountain of first class practical telling wisdom. I do not dwell on the supposed failures of his government; he has shown, I sometimes think, an almost supernatural tact in keeping the ship afloat at all, with head steady, not only going down, and now certain not to, but with proud resolute spirit, and flag flying in sight of the world, menacing and high as ever. I say, never yet captain, never ruler, never had such a perplexing dangerous task as his, the past two years. I more and more rely upon his idiomatic western genius, careless of court dress or court decorum."*

Feb 14, 1864 - James' older brother, Robert, came by today, as he's often to do. Since the death of his younger brother and James being in the military, he's taken on the care of his mother nearby. He's so caring for me. He teases me if I have a sister whom he could marry? James told me of his misfortunate accident as a child. A horse threw him upon a sharp plow, disabling him to ever have children. I know it's kept him shy of asking a wife. But I know a widow with two children of her own that would be suited for dear Robert. I've arranged for us to meet and enjoy her cooking this weekend. Hopefully they will be taken to one another.

I am most exhausted. If not, I would be consumed with worry over my beloved husband, James - having received a letter from him today was most comforting. I will most assuredly reply upon first light in the morning. As for now, I will hold this soldier's hand, as he will not make it through the night, most certainly, not another hour, in loneliness. I'm not sure which kills the body first.

Feb 16, 1864- I'm feeling burdened as I did not get to my husband's letter until late last night and posted this morning. I wrote to him of my nursing the wounded soldiers, which he already knew, hoping he will understand. He asked me to find a Sergeant from his regiment and give him word of his condition. I will try soon, today as every day, seems impossible to locate anyone in this human sea of broken bodies and mangled minds unable to even communicate their own name sometimes.

However, I was blessed, as father came through leisurely and in a pleasant mood this early afternoon and asked me aside. He expressed how Mary was finally coming to be less consumed with grief over the death of their son Willie. I, too, grieved deeply- it nearly killed them. The darkest I ever had seen him. And, rightly so. But this day, I was happy for him, as he for me, and most inquisitive about my daily life and my health. As such an admirer of poetry, he read some of mine. Such a doting daughter, I held every word of his opinion and complement in highest esteem. He actually kept one and promised to return it as soon as copied. I signed it and told him to keep it. He seemed so flattered. Yes, I detected some pride that he hides so well. But to my greatest amaze, he asked me to sign with his name, so I did, Rachel Emma Lincoln! It 'twas for the first time, ever, and brought us both great delight, so it seemed. That's when he assured me he would make known publicly his daughter after the election. That was but a seed of comparison to the love I felt from him for the first time.

Feb 20,1864 - I'm writing from my house of boarding with unimaginable joy! James is here! Father arranged a furlough. After his breakfast with other officers, the entire time we'll be together. He's more handsome than I remembered - how could that be? His kiss and embrace has left me full of inexpressible thoughts. I am full with feelings confirming our destiny. We were always to meet and marry and one day have children. I am the girl he asked to marry, and the woman he desires to lay with and wake with, perhaps even conceive with. Oh, my dear Rachel, you are hopelessly and romantically zealous!

Feb 21, 1864 – I've just kissed my beloved good bye. One night of bliss we had to so completely become one. I cannot begin to fathom tonight without him. His call to duty has overtaken him and he's needed sooner than I expected. His loyalty and duty to his men has shaped his core greater than God and country, husband and wife, mother and child.

A bond I've never witnessed to such degree, but I honor him and his decision. I must go on. I showed as little disappointment as possible. He saw through me anyway. He held me until I was at peace and left his love inside me.

DANIEL RESUMES HIS SUMMERY

And now we know that was the fateful night she conceived and confirmed the family legend. Uncanny, how she seemed to know it even then. Women are that way, you know.

Brandy changed history by being Sherman's official biographer, and rode every step of the route on the March to the Sea. It revealed truth, that it really was the Southerners who burned Ol' Dixie down. Sherman's orders were to destroy munitions plants and manufacturing which contributed to prolonging the war. Even the night they left Atlanta, after it had been completely evacuated, one such building was ordered destroyed, but the winds began to howl - as if fulfilling Sherman's decree and the fire spread relentlessly, burning almost half of the city to the ground.

As for the majority of destruction in Sherman's path to the sea, that was ordered by the Confederates, who would rather destroy their own countryside valuables than to turn them over to "those evil, invading Northerners." Sherman did systematically destroy railroads and Confederate strongholds, yet raping and pillaging were strictly propagandized rumors of Southern journalists and certainly never considered under any orders by General Sherman or his officers. There would be, however, a few disorderly and drunken Union soldiers who would steal and terrorize a few rural citizens. This is the collateral damage from any war.

Brandy was truly in his element. He also managed to have that saber given to the right family member, and with that, a passing lineage of treasure more than the saber itself, but also, a fascination to this day as to how the portal operates. He wrote of the exploits of the great train escape from Andersonville, and the follow up stories of those soldiers and their lives in prison and after the war. I could also tell that he was speaking in code by way of the language he used, knowing that I would discover his historical works. He revealed some personal tales that only I and Emo would understand. He had managed to find a telegram, in response to mine from the President, thanking Daniel Coffee for his contribution toward winning the war by accommodating General Sherman. He included a photograph of himself at the Andersonville train depot. But the one that stood out, was a photograph of Abraham Lincoln's funeral march, just as it passed what most would view as an unknown figure - a mysterious woman holding a baby child in her arms, dressed in black, watching the moment the carriage passed by with his body with intent and deep sadness. It was Rachel, holding my great grandfather. I got a chill as I sat staring at it for hours.

Emo and son put his lab on a giant old freighter ship and went searching in the Pacific for what he refers to as 'the lost great pyramid'. He still says we only have a window of time.

But there is one last chapter to my story, one I never saw coming. It made everything come full circle and completely unveil a mystery only the portal could.

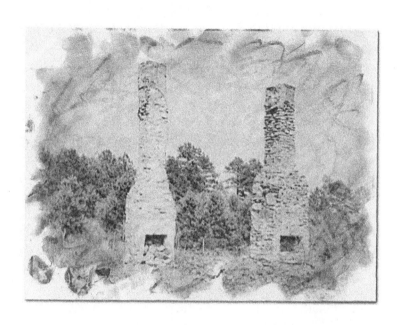

Glory Hallelujah!

GEORGIA – MANOR –BEFORE DEPARTING FOR
CALIFORNIA

Daniel has finalized the last of his packing and move
from the South, eager to get to his pregnant wife. Miss
Fitzgerald catches Daniel just as he's departing his listed
house, with the amazing memories he's left.

"Trying to get away without saying goodbye?" she
slightly teases.

"Never, I left you the most gracious letter, along with a
fine bottle of wine. Vintage 1864, I believe."

She embraces him and leaves a kiss of lipstick on his
cheek. "Of course you did. I'm going to miss our delightful
conversations. So....?" She looks at him searching for more.

He waits for her to finish. "So…?"

"…so, what's your book about and am I in it?" She still
muses at his demeanor.

"Oh, well, I think you will be quite surprised. Why,
I'd be a fool not to include such a character as you, Miss
Fitzgerald. You're a writer's dream."

"I'm relieved, and enchanted at the same time, Mr.
Daniel. Do come back and visit sometime."

Smiling, "One never knows what that 'some time' will be. Or, even what century. Goodbye, Sheila."

As he's driving away, he passes by the Waffle House. *Donna? What are the chances?* He looks over, sees her car and pulls in.

Donna dabs her eyes with a tissue while sitting in a booth by herself. Daniel approaches her with concern. "What's the matter, Donna?"

She looks up and is a little embarrassed, but still, noticeably upset. She pushes a newspaper in front of him and points to the headline.

MAN RELEASED AFTER FIFTEEN YEARS IN PRISON WRONGFULLY CONVICTED OF RAPE

"That's my husband. DNA cleared him after all these years, Mr. Daniel. I don't know how to act."

"Maybe happy? When's he coming home?" Daniel was at a loss as how to comfort her.

"Today, I just got a call from the attorney. I had no idea." She tears up again.

"Life has a strange way of coming together. That's a monumental wave of change and experience you've been through."

"Well, I never had that chance to get to know you better, I'm sure it would've come up."

"Your children will adjust. It will be a big relief to rid your family of this cloud of shame. Am I right?"

"I do want a change and I'm so happy for him. It's like a good fortune has fallen from the sky. I haven't realized it all yet… it's simply overwhelming."

"There's a great future and truth to be learned from our past, trust me. I found a treasure, you will too."

"Thank you. We're going to need it."

They exchange a hug and Daniel leaves.

Daniel is driving away to the first leg of his drive on the way to California, enjoying the countryside. After about 30 minutes he sees a hitchhiker thumbing his way as he passes. He looks in his mirror and is drawn to pull over and stop. It's a black male holding one small suit case. He gets in.

"Sho preciate ya' sir," he says in his deep country manner.

"Where you headed?" Daniel asks.

"I don't rightly know now, I just changed my mind."

Daniel and his new passenger drive off.

"You see, I was just let outta' prison after fifteen years. They let me go 'cuz I was wrongfully convicted, but I can't go home."

Daniel looks at him realizing he's Donna's husband, but keeps to himself. "Why can't you go home?"

"I'm still ashamed so bad. I know I'm a good man, but I'm scared, broke, and I have nothing to offer my family. I been a cook for all these years and I'm really good, I mean I'm *really* good. I just gotta get a start, make some money, and open a restaurant of my own. Then maybe I'll have some pride…get my family back."

Daniel fishing deeper, "That's sounds like a plan. What's your name?"

Bragging with the elegance of his full name, "Well sir, my name is Anthony Marquis De La Jacque Dupre."

The car SLAMS on its brakes in the middle of the road. Daniel throws the gear into park, puts his arm on the seat back and looks at the man with astonishment. "You got to be shittin' me!"

The stunned man tenses up. "No mistaken a name like that sir. You all right?"

Daniel looks closer at this man and shakes his head in disbelief, then glances at his leather satchel in the back seat, then back at Anthony.

He then reaches into his satchel and pulls out the map Marcus gave him and pulls it up front, along with a property title.

Feeling an epiphany, he says very slowly, "Anthony... Marcus De La Jacque Dupre, we're going to take a little detour."

Daniel makes a stop at a local hardware store just down the street, where he purchases two shovels and tosses them into the back of the suv.

It's nearing sunset over the plantation with two lone, brick chimney smokestacks. Daniel pulls up through the gate of his second property he purchased from Sheila and drives to the ruins. They both get out carrying shovels and approach the old grave site; five crosses with names mark the spot. Daniel, with map in hand, begins looking at each marker. They walk up to the only gravesite with no name and he sets down the map.

"Your ancestor left you a gift."

They both start digging as Daniel tells his loosely based story, as if it were just a legend. The sun goes slowly down the horizon, silhouetting two men, magnifying the crosses and two chimney stacks in the distance of a bygone era. Anthony is bewildered, but continues to offer his muscle in pursuit of the mystery below. The shovels make the sound of mere dirt being removed, until suddenly striking what sounds like solid metal. KERPLINK.

They hit the buried gold and jewels, far beyond what Marcus had revealed, and Daniel had nearly forgotten.

Anthony throws his shovel in the air and dances that familiar dance of freedom, shouting, "Glory Hallelujah!"

THE END

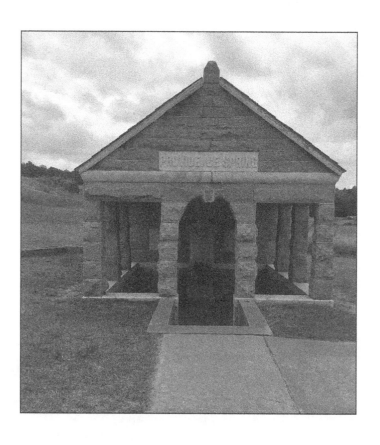

Providence Spring

ANDERSONVILLE PRISON

Prisoners turned to a narrow stream and collected rainwater for drinking as the stockade's population exploded. This stream became a quagmire of mud, stagnant water and human waste. The polluted water claimed thousands of lives, with no relief in sight for the remaining soldiers. During the second week of August 1864, 33,000 prisoners nervously watched as ominous clouds rolled in, standing in a four-walled stockade, with a muddy dirt floor, and, no covering from the elements. The rain began slowly, but quickly became a deluge. It saturated the thousands struggling for shelter underneath wool blankets and lean-tos. A flash flood destroyed a section of the stockade wall and a canon shot rang out, calling the guards to their post. The prisoners could do little but huddle together, soaking wet and cold, they began to pray aloud. A few days later, as the rain subsided, prisoners found along the deadline, in the eroded hillside, a spring of freshwater. They began using sticks and cups to reach across for water and soon a trough was built in front to funnel the clean water into the stockade, some believing that the appearance of the spring to be a miracle of God, and, hence, began calling it 'Providence Spring'. Within a month of the spring's appearance, the majority of the prisoners were evacuated to other facilities, but stories of Providence Spring quickly spread.

One of the first written accounts of the spring came from Clara Barton, and her report to the army's expedition to the site. By the early 1900's, the story emerged that lightning struck inside the prison stockade and that a spring burst forth yielding a tremendous geyser. This account reinforced the belief that the prisoners were spared through divine intervention.

In 1901, the Woman's Relief Corps and Andersonville survivors dedicated a spring house, making Providence Spring the only feature inside the stockade walls. For 150 years, Providence Spring has been an important stop among visitors to Andersonville. For previous generations, no trip to Andersonville was complete without taking a sip from the spring. Today, Providence Spring is a place where visitors can touch and feel the cool waters that eventually gave new life and hope to thousands of Americans.

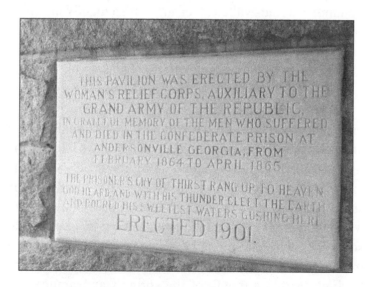

References and Influences

1. The Civil War by Ken Burns – Documentary - PBS 1990

2. Andersonville -The Last Depot by William Marvel – The University of North Carolina Press 1994

3. History of Andersonville Prison by Ovid L. Futch – University Press Florida 1968; Revised 2011

4. Southern Storm - Sherman's March to The Sea by Noah Trudeau – Harper Perennial- 2008

5. Great Maps of the Civil War by William Miller – Rutledge Hill Press 2004

6. Memoirs of General William Tecumseh Sherman –All Volumes – First Rate Publishers 2013

7. With Malice Toward None – The Life of Abraham Lincoln by Stephen B. Oats – Harper Collins Publishers 2009

8. Andersonville – Giving Up the Ghost – Collection of Prisoner's Diaries, Letters & Memoirs by Belle Grove Publishing Company 1996

9. Civil War Chronicles – American Heritage Magazine – Fall 1993

10. Wikipedia:

   Battle of Jonesborough https://en.wikipedia.org/wiki/Battle_of_Jonesborough

   Battle of Antietam https://en.wikipedia.org/wiki/Battle_of_Antietam

   Sherman's March to the Sea https://en.wikipedia.org/wiki/Sherman%27s_March_to_the_Sea

   Battle of Atlanta https://en.wikipedia.org/wiki/Battle_of_Atlanta

   Vicksburg Campaign https://en.wikipedia.org/wiki/Vicksburg_Campaign

11. The Collected Works of Abraham Lincoln by Roy P. Basler

12. Who Burned Atlanta? – NY Times by Phil Leigh – Nov 13, 2014

13. Flushed with Pride: 1850's Bathrooms https://www.livescience.com/17972-1850s-bathroom-preserved.html

14. 31st Regiment ILL https://civilwar.illinoisgenweb.org/reg_html/031_reg.html

15. 52nd Regiment ILL https://civilwar.illinoisgenweb.org/reg_html/052_reg.html

16. Solar Flares and Earth's Electromagnetic Field. http://cse.ssl.berkeley.edu/SegwayEd/lessons/exploring_magnetism/in_Solar_Flares/index.html

17. Sherman's Inability to Liberate the South's Most Notorious Prison https://ehistory.osu.edu/ articles/shermans-inability-liberate-souths-most-notorious-prison

18. Andersonville National Historic Site Georgia – National Park Service - Andersonville National Cemetery
National Prisoner of War Museum, 496 Cemetery Road, Andersonville, GA 31711

19. Handwritten Diary and Memoirs – Charles Orr – Author's Great Great Uncle

20. Handwritten Letters to his wife 1863-1864 – James H. Miller – Author's Great - Great Grandfather

21. The Source Field Investigations by David Wilcock – Penguin Group 2011

22. HeartMath Institute: The Coherent Heart – Heart-Brain Interactions, Psychophysiological Coherence, and the Heart's Electromagnetic Field by Rollin McCraty, Ph.D.; Mike Atkinson, Dana Tomasino, Raymond Trevor Bradly. Ph.D. 1998-2003

23. Heart Intelligence: Connecting with the Intuitive Guidance of the Heart by Doc Childre, Howard Martin, Deborah Rozman and Rollin McCraty – Waterfront Press – HeartMath 2016

24. Civil War Poetry and Prose by Walt Whitman – Dover Publications 1995

25. Civil War Poetry an Anthology by Pau; Negri – Dover Press 1997

MUSIC and ARTWORK

I Am A Rebel Soldier – A traditional folk song during the Civil War from Southern Appalachia - author unknown.

When Johnny Comes Marching Home by Patrick Gilmore -1863

Moonlight Sonata by Ludwig van Beethoven

Sarah's Theme by Michael Meyer

Artwork page 192 Banjo Player by Charles Ethan Porter 1847-1923

Cover Design by Michael Meyer; Photography by Rene Victor Bidez, Fayetteville, GA.

Charcoal Illustrations by Vivid Images Productions

PROCLAMATIONS

During his presidency Abraham Lincoln issued a total of nine proclamations of prayer, fasting, or thanksgiving. The first one was issued on August 12, 1861, in response to a request from Congress. Source for the text of documents: *The Collected Works of Abraham Lincoln*. https://quod.lib. umich.edu/l/lincoln/ Roy P. Basler and his editorial staff.

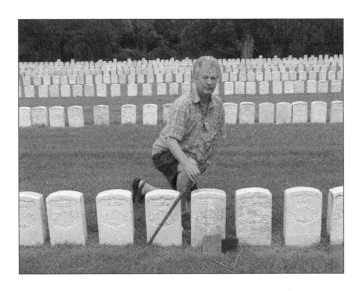

Michael Meyer,
Author, Family Historian

Michael Meyer currently lives in Fayetteville, Georgia. He runs Hollywood South Accommodations, an Airbnb for the film industry and local studios, and writes original and adapted screenplays. Some of his notable works are *From Mafia Boss to the Cross* and *Behold the Whirlwind*.

A current listing of his projects can be seen at <u>www. vividimagesproductions.com</u>.

CPSIA information can be obtained
at www.ICGtesting.com
Printed in the USA
LVHW05205315091 9
631103LV00004B/57/P